How to Afford Veterinary Care

Without Mortgaging the Kids

Common Sense and Money Saving Advice From an Old, Country Vet

Dr. James L. Busby D.V.M.

Cover and Layout by Laura Kuznia
Photography Monty Draper

www.oldcountryvet.com
info@oldcountryvet.com

Dr. Jim L Busby D.V.M.
Old Country Vet
1726 Jefferson Ave SW
Bemidji MN, 56601

Old Country Vet World Wide Website Address is:
www.oldcountryvet.com

Arrow Printing
1375 Washington Ave S
Bemidji MN, 56601

Arrow Printing World Wide Website Address is:
www.arrowprintinginc.com

Special thanks to Marty Busby, Suzi Ross

Printed in the U.S.A.

Thank You
Marty and Barb

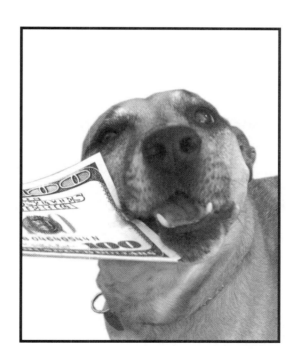

Introduction

This is dedicated to Barb, who motivated me with her off the cuff suggestion that I put my honest and experienced, money saving advice into a book, and to my wife Marty, who gave me tremendous support in my effort.

This book started off basically as a result of a conversation with a client who lives 240 miles away in the Twin Cities. Her family had a summer cabin in the area and she found her way to me by talking to some locals. In our conversation she complained about the expense of veterinary care in her area. When I pointed out numerous procedures she had paid for that were, in my opinion, unnecessary, she indicated that putting my knowledge and honest recommendations in book form would be a good idea. I have tried to do just that. I have experienced a growing anger with the way the veterinary profession has evolved over the past decade or so and it felt good to put my feelings down on paper. What follows is my advice. This is what I tell my clients. It will give you a second opinion on a menagerie of things concerning your pet and it comes from someone who has been actively and successfully treating dogs and cats for 40 years. I'm sure that what I have written will greatly upset the rank and file of the profession but I'm 65 years old and really don't feel loyalty to those who I consider to be both unethical and outright fraudulent in the way they practice. You can judge for your self after reading this book who are the good ones and who aren't.

Table of Content

Part 2: Miscellaneous Advice

These are all examples of how the modern day veterinarian can mislead the public under the guise of being a caring, animal loving doctor wanting only what's best for your pet. I feel that almost all of the above procedures are either often unnecessary or a total rip off to increase the bottom line. I will take each of the above, tell you why I say that and enlighten you as to how you can eliminate the unnecessary and unwarranted procedures. I'm sure you can use the money as well as your veterinarian.

ALSO INCLUDED-----
Miscellaneous comments: My 40 years of experience with dealing with both client's pets and over a dozen of my own. Information and tricks of the trade on what and how best to do it.

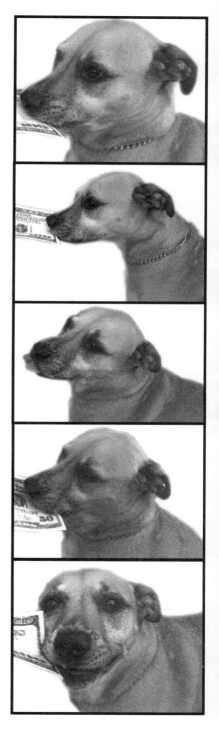

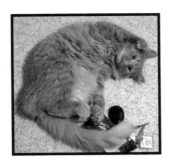

Preface

An elderly gentleman came into my outpatient clinic a while ago for his first visit with two very geriatric, mid sized terriers. He wanted the nails clipped and for me to check the anal glands on the "younger" 15 year old. There was a dime sized, slightly reddened swelling just below the animal's rectum that at first glance looked like an infected anal gland. It turned out to be too centrally located for an infected gland and was not sore to the touch, which an infection would have been. Upon questioning, the owner stated the swelling had been present for at least a year. Then the story unfolded. He had taken the animal to a different clinic where the doctor had expressed great alarm over the lump. She strongly pressed for its surgical removal on the grounds it would soon interfere with the animal's ability to pass its feces. Urine and blood tests were run and then, on the pretence that she thought the "cancer" might have spread to the kidneys, she insisted on a $700 test to evaluate this. When three weeks passed without hearing from the clinic, he called and demanded to know what they found out. She called the lab where the test had been sent and informed him that the results were inconclusive. But she had good news: Another test would be needed but this one would only cost $150. That's when he decided on a second opinion.

The lump was small. It had been there for over a year without appreciably changing in size, which meant there was no way it could in the foreseeable future interfere with the animal's ability to defecate. In 40 years I've never seen an external growth interfere with defecation ability. Internal yes-external no. It wasn't hurting the dog. In fact the animal didn't even know it was there. There were two choices: live with it or remove it. I told him to just watch it and save any heroic surgery for the time when it started to enlarge enough to be a problem, if ever, because the dog would probably live another year or so and die of non-related old age causes.

When I asked him the reason the other clinic gave for spending so much of his money testing to see if there was a chance the supposed cancer had possibly spread to the kidneys, he related that they had to see the test results before they could tell him. If the dog had tested positive, there wouldn't have been a damn thing they could have done about changing the progression of cancer in the kidneys in a 15 year old dog without horrendous involvement. And of course there is the small matter of many thousands of dollars that would have been involved in surgical removal of a kidney, the extreme risk of the surgery to the old animal and probable chemotherapy afterwards that had never been discussed with the owner before so foolishly wasting his money. They never considered asking him if he would have been agreeable to this, which he wouldn't have been. Of course then they couldn't have made any money playing doctor. ASK QUESTIONS BEFORE YOU GET SUCKED INTO SOME EXPENSIVE QUAGMIRE LIKE THIS. Veterinarians today seem to assume that they have the OK to run every test and perform any and every procedure on your animal they can think of unless you tell them differently. Then they usually get irate and try to shame you for being a non loving pet owner. Remember that each test will probably lead to something much more expensive. Even if money isn't short, question thoroughly before proceeding with each step.

II

I have been a practicing veterinarian since 1966. My father, uncle and great grand father were also veterinarians. I have enjoyed my profession and never regretted this choice for my life's work, but sadly, I would never enter the profession today, if I had to practice in the way things are currently done. I feel the profession has slowly turned from what was once an honest, caring one to a situation, where many clinics and doctors are interested more in the bottom line, than what is necessary and best for your pet. Every client through the door is just someone else to try to push as many procedures and services on as the pet owner will tolerate, in order to generate as large a cash return as possible. All under the guise of doing only what's best for his or her beloved animal. And, when your trusted doctor says this is what is absolutely needed to maintain the health of your pet, you believe it's necessary. But many people are slowly coming to the realization that a lot of what's recommended is actually unnecessary, "make work" procedures. Having spent 40 years in the profession, I can tell you that, sadly, this is often unfortunately true.

It is recommended that each individual see his or her doctor yearly for an annual checkup, see the dentist twice yearly for cleaning and exams, and as you get older pap smears, mammograms, prostrate tests and checks, colon exams, cholesterol tests and a basket full of other diagnostic measures are recommended. If insurance pays the cost, many but not all will comply with at least some of these. Those without insurance pretty much forget about it as the cost is too prohibitive in light of all their other expenses, which are rising much faster than their income. Your pet's medical costs are almost always directly right out of your pocket and even those with animal insurance find it often saves hardly more than what the policy costs. I am going to tell you just what I feel you should do to keep your animal as healthy as possible, without causing strain on your budget or incurring undue risk and pain to your pet. They don't like needles any more than you do. Twice a year dental exams, yearly health checks, repeated vaccinations, tests for heartworm, Lyme disease, intestinal parasites, Giardia, leukemia, heart and blood are all recommended. Are all these necessary? Just like the recommendations for you listed above, these may be of some benefit in diagnosing a few disease problems but are almost never justifiable in households even without limited budgets. The vast majority of animals will stay healthy and live long normal lives without the extra expense these would entail. Many of these animal preventative measures fall under what is called "wellness checks" and are geared, at least in my mind, more to keeping the clinic's finances healthy rather than the pets.

Even though the modern day veterinarian is trying to pattern the treatment of animals in somewhat the same way that human medicine treats people, there will always be a fundamental difference. In human medicine there is almost always a "no holds barred" attitude that cannot be justified for animals, except for the monetarily affluent. People either have insurance for themselves or they have the knowledge that no emergency clinic will turn away anyone in need, even though they can't pay. In veterinary medicine you pay all costs yourself and often up front. Pet insurance is pretty much not cost effective. In this modern world, hundreds and sometimes thousands of dollars in unexpected veterinary costs can be an intolerable burden. Added to that is the great variation in degree to which people hold their pets. Many consider them to be absolutely dear and would mortgage their very soul in order to attempt to save them. Then there are those on the other side of the coin who tolerate animals as a pet but think "for God's sake it's only a dog", when medical costs pass a bare minimum. And in the middle are those on a fixed income, who dearly love the company of their pet, but yet can hardly afford to pay anything extra in treatment and care.

What you read below is the absolute same advice and CHOICES that I give my clients. It is based on 40 year's experience coupled with current known facts and treatment results. It is my advice and mine alone. Everything evolves with time and nothing is absolute, but this advice is knowledgeable and basic. I will point out what I consider necessary for disease treatment and prevention and what I think can be eliminated for economy purposes, without unnecessarily jeopardizing your dear animal's life. I feel you should always have the choice between minimum treatment and the sky's the limit sort of thing. Most veterinarians shoot for the latter and almost never mention the first, even though minimum is often all that's needed.

Part 1

Many Veterinarians Recommend most or all of these Procedures

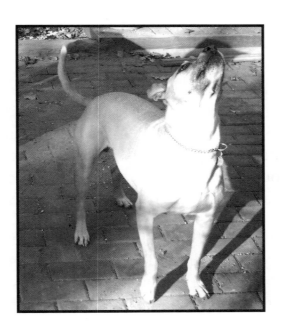

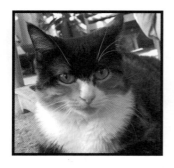

Chapter 1

ANNUAL OR REPEATING VACCINATIONS
EVERY TWO YEARS

For many, many years it was routine for veterinarians to recommend yearly vaccinations for distemper, parvo virus and rabies in dogs and distemper and rabies in cats and absolutely insist your animal was in dire jeopardy if this advice was not followed. This practice apparently originated because the vaccine manufacturer said it was necessary. No one questioned it. Who knows more about the vaccination duration than the company who makes it? You can trust them. Right? NOT NECESSARILY!!!

Consider how often your family physician recommends vaccinations for your children. They receive one inoculation during early childhood and that lasts them basically for life. Why do you suppose four legged animals are any different? They apparently aren't. It doesn't take a rocket scientist to figure out that a vaccine manufacturer isn't going to go to great lengths to offer research saying its vaccine needs to be given only once or twice during the life of a pet when sales can be made yearly. Remember veterinarians reap the same monetary benefit with repeat inoculations, so most of them are not going to rock the boat either.

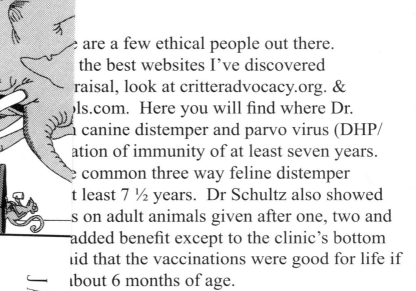

...e are a few ethical people out there. ...the best websites I've discovered ...raisal, look at critteradvocacy.org. & ...ls.com. Here you will find where Dr. ...a canine distemper and parvo virus (DHP/ ...ation of immunity of at least seven years. ...e common three way feline distemper ...t least 7 ½ years. Dr Schultz also showed ...s on adult animals given after one, two and ...added benefit except to the clinic's bottom ...iid that the vaccinations were good for life if ...ibout 6 months of age.

...nimal Hospital Association (AAHA) ...a recommendation of repeating these ...ee years BUT this was a compromise ...iere was no data to suggest three years - ...led out of the air and the organization let it be known that they felt the shots were good for a lot longer -- probably life. The American Veterinary Medical Association (AVMA) also said that "There is no scientific data to support the annual administration of MLV (modified live virus) vaccines." Then they also folded and left it up to the discretion of the veterinarian. (Fox guarding the hen house sort of thing).

From everything I've read, there have never been any studies showing the need to repeat distemper/parvo on dogs or distemper on cats after they were given to an animal 6 months or older. There HAVE been several studies showing the shots are good for at least 7 years and in all probability for life. There are basically no scientific grounds for repeating every 1 to 3 years if ever.

Between 6 and 12 weeks of age, repeating the DHP/PV vaccination does have merit for this reason: The maternal antibodies the nursing animal gets from the mother's milk protect it during the nursing period and for a short time afterwards. These antibodies are passive—they don't reproduce themselves in the young animal and come only from the mother. When nursing stops, they are soon gone. The antibodies not only offer protection against the diseases in question but, since they can't differentiate between the weakened and very similar virus and bacteria in the vaccines, will destroy them also. The vaccine needs to be repeated until a time when the maternal antibodies are gone (very close to 100% gone at 14 weeks of age) and then the young animal will be stimulated to produce its own active, "probably lifelong" antibodies. The rub is that almost all veterinarians insist on repeating these vaccinations over and over again throughout the life of the pet. Never forget how often they need to be given to you or your kids. ONCE!!!

Any vaccination given after 13 or 14 weeks of age to a pet is considered its first adult shot. It's probably good for life, but repeating the series in a year would certainly cinch the deal. Additional inoculations after that are apparently a waste of your money and even a possible health risk to your pet. Drawing blood to run a titer (titer explained in chapter 16) to see if the animal has adequate protection is NOT a good investment. The AVMA itself stated that an animal's titer is not an accurate indication of protection. The ONLY adequate test is resistance to actual disease exposure.

For forty years I recommended that my clients vaccinate their puppies at six weeks with DHP/PV, repeat with a PV booster at nine weeks and give the adult shots (DHP/PV & rabies) at 13 to 14 weeks of age. There is never a guarantee in anything in life except supposedly death and taxes but this worked 100% for me for 40 years. I always recommended a repeat of the adult shots in 12 months. After that I'm convinced it's a waste of money. Rabies vaccination is the only ringer. For legality purposes the government demands repeat vaccinations every three years. The first one is repeated in one year but then not more often then every three years. Any oftener than that is another example of unethical veterinarians deceiving you for profit. This is true for both cats and dogs.

There are a dozen other things you can vaccinate your cat or dog for. I have never pushed them because I don't feel they were justified. Kennel cough and Lyme vaccinations are two common ones. I personally think they are both very over hyped. The first is a viral bronchitis (cough-- much like the cough you would get with the flu) that I have never seen a case of. The literature talks like it is almost always mild and self limiting, so why the big push to vaccinate? The second is very rare and easily treatable. No big deal! I've talked to the University of Minnesota Veterinary Diagnostic Lab repeatedly and they say they see only about one case of Lyme disease a year and have never seen a fatality with it.

After an animal reaches 13 or 14 weeks of age I'm convinced there is NO BENEFIT in giving a series of vaccinations. One gives all the stimulation necessary according to people who know and are honest about it. Animals are basically the same whether they are two or four legged. When someone tells you that vaccinations need to be repeated over and over again, think how often they need to be repeated on you or your children. Once and that's it for life. The reason flu vaccinations are repeated each year is because a NEW virus appears almost yearly and a different vaccine is needed to immunize you to prevent a totally new brand of flu. If the virus didn't change, the vaccination received the year before or many years before would still be adequate.

Some statements I've found at critteradvocacy.org:
Lepto vaccinations---the risk of side effects out weigh benefits.
Giardia vaccinations are not recommended.
FIV (feline immuno-suppressive virus) vaccination not recommended
Ringworm vaccinations are not recommended.
Chlamydia vaccinations are not recommended.
Kennel cough vaccination protects against only 2 of over 8 different causes.
FIP (feline infectious peritonitis) vaccination not recommended.
Corona virus vaccination not recommended.

Canine influenza (flu) has been in the news as of late and has received a lot of hype. Here is some input from the veterinary journals and newsletters: A Dr. Brad Fenwick, vice president for research and professor of infectious disease at Virginia-Maryland Regional College of Veterinary Medicine has treated hundreds of racing greyhounds with the disease. He probably has as much experience with it as anybody. Here is a quote he made in the article in DVM Newsmagazine of November 2005: "I'm afraid the media hype may prescribe yet ANOTHER UNWARRANTED VACCINE in veterinary medicine." He feels the deaths were due to inadequate antibiotic treatment in more severe cases which allowed the animals to develop a bacterial pneumonia. He said, "Because canine influenza is mild, half of all infected dogs will show no clinical signs. The average pet owner might not even recognize them. This is being over hyped."

REMEMBER THIS when, in a couple of years, your veterinarian is going to tell you "Fluffy" has to be vaccinated because I will absolutely guarantee you a vaccine will come on the market. And I bet it will be required twice the first year and annually forever after.

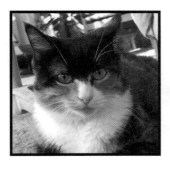

Notes

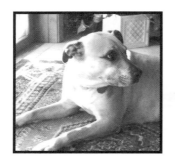

Chapter 2

YEARLY TESTING FOR HEARTWORM

Heartworm testing and prevention has been a money maker for veterinary clinics for years. Veterinarians imply that it's dangerous to give the preventative to an infected dog. I am NOT aware of a product currently being used as a monthly preventive that can't be given to a dog infected with Dirofilaria immitis, which is the scientific name for heartworm. Doses of ivermectin (the active ingredient in Heartgard), at approximately 40 times as strong as in the preventive, are given to dogs following treatment for heartworm to remove the microfilaria that are still circulating in the blood stream. (Microfilaria are tiny larva-like "babies" of the heartworm that circulate in the blood and two or three are sucked up by a mosquito when it feeds on a dog—these are later injected into another dog when a mosquito bites it weeks later after maturing in the insect). Also a little known piece of information that few veterinarians will volunteer is that Heartgard, or its active ingredient ivermectin, if given once a month to a known infected dog for 18 months will cure an animal of the infection. Cage confinement is not recommended with this treatment method.

Apparently veterinarians don't want you to cure a possibly infected dog yourself. They want to test first so they can make a big deal out of it and charge you for a treatment! So is a pretest necessary before administering the monthly preventive? Not as

8

far as the health of the dog is concerned, but it's a real boon to the clinic's financial picture. Besides using an often overlooked commodity called common sense, if the preventative is any good at all, and they are all excellent, why does one need to test every year before re-giving the medication?

One of the reasons made to justify yearly testing, besides the deception that your animal might be harmed if the preventative is inadvertently given to an infected dog, is because there may have been a few suspected cases of heartworm in dogs that were supposedly on the preventative. Apparently they want to use your money through yearly testing to try to determine if this is true and clarify what products work best.

Outside dogs get a lot more mosquito exposure than house pets. A single infected mosquito carries 1 to 3 potential worms. It takes repeated bites from infected mosquitoes to reach a level of infection that will show symptoms. I remember reading once where the American Heartworm Society implied that a few worms in a healthy dog were probably not clinically significant and yearly testing was hard to justify. They have since been PERSUADED to change their recommendation to call for yearly tests and treat all levels of infection. (The board is composed solely of veterinarians—kind of like the fox guarding the hen house). Blood tests will diagnose an infection of as few as one or two worms and it is very debatable that an infection rate that slight even necessitates treatment. The adult worm has a life span of about 5 years and then will die of old age. If you knew your animal was infected, I would offer the option to put it on Heartgard or the equivalent once a month for at least a year instead of the much more expensive in clinic treatment, which would cost many hundreds of dollars more.

Heart worm infection is not necessarily a kiss of death. The worms are a physical impediment to the passage of blood to the lungs. The more worms present in the arteries carrying this blood, the more difficulty in blood passage. When there is a large enough glob of worms present, the animal will start to show a low grade but persistent throat clearing cough especially with exercise. When your animal has this many worms, you have a real problem. Most diagnosed cases are in animals having too few worms to show symptoms.

Cats can also get heart worm but in my experience it is rare. Supposedly the symptoms are more acute and severe. If your cat spends a lot of time outside, it is probably a good idea to put it on the preventative also.

A Money Saving Tip: There are two cat sizes and four dog sizes based directly on weight of the animal. The price for each different size is almost the same. If you have a smaller animal, purchase the larger size and break the tablet into halves or quarters and cut your cost accordingly. This idea can also be a good money saver for people who take a lot of prescription pills. Most drug manufacturers charge the same for all sizes of the same tablet. Ask your doctor if it's feasible to have the next larger size prescribed, get a pill splitter to cut it in half and probably save half on your prescription costs.

Another Option to Save Money on Heartworm is: Ivermectin (the active ingredient in Heartgard) is available as an over the counter wormer for large animals. It can be bought without a prescription over the internet or from a farm supply store. It comes in a 50 cc (ml) bottle of 1% solution. You want the liquid (not the paste) that states 1 cc (ml) worms 110 pounds of animal. It costs less than $1.00 a ml. One ml will prevent heart worm in about 30 one hundred pound dogs for a month. Compared to Heartgard, it is MUCH more concentrated and obviously a lot cheaper. 1/10th of a ml contains as much ivermectin as is found in THREE Heartgard doses for dogs weighing 100 pounds. It is injected into hogs and cattle to eliminate intestinal parasites. For someone with larger numbers of bigger dogs, this could be both an inexpensive general wormer plus heartworm preventive. There is a possibility of side effects when used at the general worming dose (not heartworm prevention dose) but it is remote, except for collies and herding dogs. It is probably safer than your taking any over the counter pain medication for a prolonged period of time. Animals that get a reaction have to have an inherited weakness and collies are much more likely to have this.

　　　1. 1/10th of a ml (cc) is the intestinal worming dose when given for each 11 lbs. of dog or cat. In pets it is given by MOUTH--NOT INJECTED. This is for intestinal worms (roundworms, hookworms etc.). Heartworm prevention requires no more than 1/10th that much (1/10th ml per 100 lbs) given monthly just like Heartgard. This dose is at the stronger end that Heartgard considers being safe and should insure your animal DOESN'T get infected. Technically this dose is 10 mcg per pound. The small dog dose of Heartgard goes as high as 35 mcg per pound of dog. A reaction isn't expected in a susceptible animal until given a dose just over 60 mcg per pound and this SHOULD be a mild reaction with the animal back to normal within 24 hours. I've read that 60 mcg per pound of body weight has been given to Collies that were known to be sensitive without problems.

2. DO NOT USE THIS INTESTINAL WORMING DOSE IN COLLIES OR HERDING DOGS WITH FOUR WHITE FEET. The above heartworm dose would be OK.

3. It is not particularly toxic in normal animals. As an example I've used it numerous times to treat demodectic mange in young dogs at a dose three times what is needed to treat intestinal worms; (1 ml per 35 lbs.) DAILY for three months. This is 300 mcg per pound. An animal has to be born with a couple of the right recessive genes to suffer a reaction from it. If these genes are present, a coma may develop if given a dose of approximately 1/10th ml (cc) per 20 lbs. or more according to the original manufacturers. (cc and ml. are the same).

SUMMARY
*Ivermectin 1 % injectable solution in 50 ml bottle.
*1/10th ml orally per 11 lbs. treats intestinal worms. The risk of having the recessive genes in dogs other than collies or herding dogs is about one in 5000 or less. Most human prescriptions carry more risk of complications. Since ability to react is inherited, if a dog did have a problem, others from the same litter could be at risk also.

*1/10th ml orally per 20 lbs SHOULD be safe in any animal but only 1/10th ml per 100 lbs. is needed to prevent heartworms. Don't use over this amount in collies or herding dogs with 4 white feet.

*You would need a 1 cc (ml) tuberculin syringe to measure this small of an amount accurately.

*How to try to test if a dog would react for intestinal worming: (worming dose for 50 lbs is 0.5 ml)

50 pound dog: Start with 0.2 ml. first day.
Next day give 0.25 ml.
Next day give 0.3 ml. (remote chance)
Next day give 0.35 ml. (reaction expected here)
Next day give 0.4 ml.
Next day give 0.45 ml.
Next day give 0.5 ml. (This is worming dose-- the dog obviously didn't react.)

If at any time dog acts uncoordinated—stop!

This would signify that the animal will have no problem. Obviously, if at any time during the testing period the dog becomes wobbly, don't give it any more. The one time I used this test on a Collie pup, it reacted but was back to normal the next day. This method was told me by the manufacturers. Remember, when I treated demodectic mange, I would give 1 ml per 35 lbs. daily for 3 months. It has a high degree of safety in normal dogs.

For any adventuresome souls who might be interested, 1cc syringes can be purchased over the internet. Get one without needle attached. 1 % ivermectin can be diluted in 100% propylene glycol, which is also available. Mixing 1 ml of ivermectin with 3 ml of propylene glycol will dilute it to 1/4th as strong. 1/10th ml of this dilution should be safe for any 25 pound dog for monthly heartworm prevention. Diluting 1 cc ivermectin in 7 cc propylene glycol makes it 1/8th as strong. 1/10 ml should be safe for a 12 pound animal for heartworm prevention.

This information above is to enable you to safely use a large animal form of ivermectin to prevent heartworm and also as a general wormer if you so desire. It would be quite an economical alternative but you must understand the simple basics in order to use it properly.

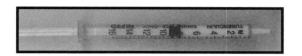

Do not use the side of the syringe marked with a letter M (by the point) this is the back side.

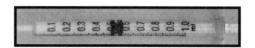

Use the front side of syringe. This picture shows a 1 ml syringe filled half full or 0.5 ml of ivermectin. (ml and cc mean the same thing)

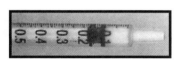

This is an enlargement of a 1 cc (ml) syringe shows the syringe filled to the 0.1 ml mark. This amount of concentrated 1% ivermectin would be safe according to the experts for any dog over 30 lbs to prevent heartworm.

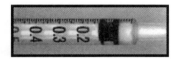

This picture is showing the 1 ml syringe filled to 1/2 of the 0.1 ml.

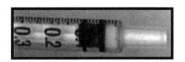

This picture is showing the 1 ml syringe filled to 1/3 of 0.1 ml. This amount of concentrated 1% ivermectin would contain about 333 ug of wormer. When you try to measure this small of an amount of a concentrated wormer, there is a lot more room for error if you are off even a little.

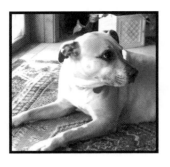

Notes

_____
_____
_____
_____
_____
_____
_____
_____
_____
_____
_____
_____
_____
_____
_____
_____
_____
_____
_____
_____
_____
_____
_____
_____
_____
_____

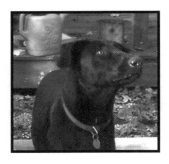

Chapter 3

TESTING FOR LYME DISEASE

I am personally aware of several veterinary practices that push Lyme disease testing for every normal dog that enters the clinic and repeating it on a yearly basis. Is this good advice? NOT IN MY JUDGEMENT!!! The American Veterinary Medical Association published an article in its journal in November of 2003 stating that you can't diagnose Lyme disease based on test results, because any where from 25% to 85% of dogs can test positive and, when these animals were followed for several years, they were no more likely to come down with the disease than the animals that tested negative. In other words, the test was worthless! Would you be surprised if I told you that these clinics were then treating the dogs that tested positive even though they showed no symptoms and were healthy and happy? In my opinion this is just another way to generate income from the unsuspecting public. I feel something like this should be considered unethical.

My experience with Lyme disease has been this: I saw five cases about 1990. They all responded very quickly to an inexpensive old antibiotic called tetracycline with complete recovery. I haven't seen a case since. It is a real threat to people but, at least in my area, dogs have seemed to learn to live with it. Obviously there is a lot of exposure, which is the reason so many dogs have blood titers (titer explained in chapter 16) and test positive, but they just don't seem to develop disease symptoms. I have had several medical people tell me that the human test gives a lot of positives in people also, who never come down with the disease.

Lyme disease in dogs is basically a single, progressing into multiple leg lameness. The vast majority of single leg pain is due to minor injury just like you'd see when you sprain your leg. If a second leg is involved, then Lyme should be considered. When I would suspect a possible case of the tick carried disease, I would treat the animal for five days with both anti-inflammatory medication to treat a possible injury and an antibiotic effective for Lyme disease. The animal would respond to treatment. If Lyme disease was the culprit, the lameness would return with a vengeance a few days after treatment stopped. Dramatic response to the antibiotic alone in just a couple more days of additional treatment was pretty good conformation of the disease and 5 weeks of continuous treatment eliminated the problem totally. The test would have proved nothing except that the dog carried a titer as do countless others that don't show symptoms. Some veterinarians will automatically run a Lyme test on any dog that limps. Since a positive test could NEVER even remotely be considered a conclusive diagnosis of Lyme disease, don't waste your money. Possibly even consider getting a different vet who is more attuned to the facts.

Should you vaccinate for it? I don't vaccinate my three dogs. The University of Minnesota Veterinary Diagnostic Laboratory through the end of 2004 told me they only see about one case a year and have never seen a fatality from it. They also implied the test is pretty much a waste. If you do vaccinate, the manufacturer recommends two initial vaccinations and then an annual one forever after. Knowing that this was the identical recommendation given for decades for distemper and parvo virus by the same companies, does this make you mildly suspicious of the need for so many repeat inoculations?

Parting words on Lyme disease: I've just read that a survey of the 27 veterinary colleges in the U.S. showed that 19 DIDN'T recommend even vaccinating for it. The other 8 would if the owner requested but didn't stress the need. Serious complications attributed to Lyme disease are rare and have often been blamed on THE VACCINE rather than exposure to the disease itself. My recommendation would be to forget about vaccinating for it since it is so rare and easy to treat. I've also read several times that although antibiotic treatment will rapidly cure symptoms, it will NOT eliminate the organism from the animal. HOW ABOUT THAT? Don't treat a dog just because it tests positive and a limp is far from qualifying as a positive symptom of Lyme disease. A limp is usually only symptomatic of a sprain and your vet ought to know better.

I also learned at a recent conference that there has not yet been a confirmed case of Lyme disease affecting a dog's kidneys. A couple of POSSIBLE cases (not proven) have been hyped up to the point that a positive Lyme test (remember how worthless this was in diagnosing anything) is justification to run kidney function tests and any irregularity here results in treatment for the disease. A worthless Lyme test leads to a kidney test which looks for a disease that has never been diagnosed and this leads to a treatment that probably won't eliminate the bacteria from a dog's system!!! If this isn't an oscar winning performance of wasting a client's money without just cause, I'd like a better example.

20

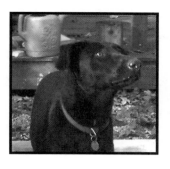

Notes

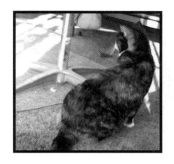

Chapter 4

TESTING FOR LEUKEMIA

Leukemia testing for cats is pushed pretty much nation wide. Is this good advice? I don't feel it's justified and here's why. Leukemia in cats is caused by a virus so it can spread from one animal to another, although the spread is slow and may take years. Also, some animals that were positive to the test may expel the virus and test negative in following years. Since the disease is viral caused, it is not considered treatable or curable. In my opinion and using good old common sense again, the only place where the test has any merit is when performed on a cat about to be purchased. If it's positive, you don't want to bring it into the house. Testing a healthy animal as a routine measure serves no purpose because you will not want to destroy a beloved pet that may never show symptoms. Even in a multiple cat household, where one animal has become sick and was confirmed to have the disease, testing the rest will pinpoint any other carriers, but your options are again to destroy them or let them live as long as possible.

Remember that not all positive cats will die and there is no treatment to prevent a carrier from coming down with the disease. If you are not willing to destroy the animal, how has the test benefited you? It will benefit the clinic though, because it will give them cause to insist on a thorough and expensive check up every few months in order to monitor your pet's health. I certainly would not choose to euthanise my cat under those circumstances. All you can do is vaccinate the rest in order to try to prevent them from becoming infected. Veterinarians insist on testing all cats before vaccinating. This is mostly a cover your rear move because the vaccine will not protect a positive animal. I compromised by telling my clients that it would not protect an infected cat but, since it cost more to test than to vaccinate, I recommended forgetting the test and just vaccinating. I told them, if the animals lived a year or two without coming down with symptoms, they were probably out of danger.

A small percentage of vaccinated cats develop a very nasty, life threatening cancer at the site of vaccination. I don't think any one is positive just which vaccine is the culprit but the leukemia shot is at the top of the list for suspects. The vaccine manufacturer is again recommending two initial vaccinations and annual thereafter. This plays like a broken record. Remember Dr. Schultz's findings that repeat vaccinations on adult animals provided no added benefit? If your cat never spends any time outside, it is never going to be exposed. Don't vaccinate. A multiple cat household, whose animals spend a lot of time outside, are more likely to have someone exposed and bring the problem home to someone else. Here vaccination is a better investment. It's a common sense judgment if you should vaccinate and again how often.

This is one vaccine that might carry bad side effects especially if repeated too frequently.

New Information: Leukemia vaccine has officially been classified as a carcinogenic (cancer causing) agent by the state of California. And it is felt that almost 90% of cats develop a natural resistance to leukemia whether vaccinated or not by one year of age. Symptoms occurring in animals up to seven years of age are probably a result of exposure between birth and one year. 22,000 cats are reported to die yearly in this country from vaccine induced cancers. All vaccines seem to carry SOME risk for cats. Knowing this, I would be reluctant to recommend vaccinating an animal more than once for leukemia after reaching one year of age.

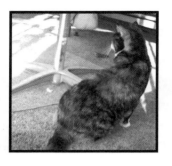

Notes

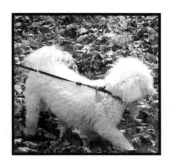

Chapter 5

TESTING AND VACCINATING FOR GIARDIA

Giardia is a much hyped problem that I think is way overblown. It is a tiny parasite that can live in the intestine and is found in many normal dogs that never show any symptoms. The only problem I have personally felt was caused by this parasite in 40 years of practice has possibly been an off again-on again soft and slimy stool. It's something that often bothers the owner more than the dog. I get just as much benefit for a cure by having the owner add oat bran (a cereal in the breakfast food section- an excellent source of quality fiber) to the diet every day rather than using a medicinal treatment, like the wormer Pancur, which costs a lot more. Oat bran both firms up loose stools and softens those those are too hard. Works on people too and also lowers cholesterol!

Most cases of diarrhea will self correct without treatment, particularly in adult dogs, but if your animal develops a severe diarrhea that persists for several days, especially if the animal shows secondary symptoms of not being quite up to par, then you can choose to see your veterinarian. If the stool shows any shape at all (piles up a little rather than runs) I don't consider it to be a serious problem. If this softness persists and it bothers you, first try to control it with diet change especially by adding oat bran or changing back to a diet that you know your pet can tolerate. I have never seen any harm from simple human anti-diarrheas purchased over the counter. Remember that if your dog is only a fraction of your weight; treat accordingly.

There is a vaccine for Giardia, but the American Animal Hospital Association does NOT recommend it. There is also a test for the problem, but I consider it to be in the same category as the Lymes test. A lot of normal animals will test positive so does the test actually have any benefit? And a positive test on a dog with diarrhea is not proof that giardia is the cause. Just treating diarrhea symptoms has been a very effective common sense tactic in my 40 years of practice. TRY THAT FIRST and reserve the expensive laboratory work for just the few unresponsive cases. Most loose stools in esp. older dogs are directly related to sudden changes in diet. And most are self correcting. If common sense home treatment, diet changes or a few days time don't correct the problem, then proceed to medical help, especially if the animal seems to be affected through slowed activity. Just don't panic. You get diarrhea also on occasion. Do you rush to the doctor when that happens or do you use common sense? Approach your animal's problem the same way.

I just read that rice and chicken broth were as effective as anything for simple diarrhea in people. Try it on your pet. New puppies often get a looseness of the stools shortly after arrival. Rushing to the vet will immediately transform into a large expense. Again use common sense. If the puppy feels good, is eating and drinking and NOT pooping more than every few hours, give it a little time to correct. Feeding a bland diet the first few days and/ or feeding nothing but the same dog food it had been used to will often prevent this. I've known more cases where the veterinarian would make a mountain out of this molehill and rack up a tremendous bill for an emotional owner. Sometimes coccidiosis will flare up under the stress of being shipped to a new home. This is very easily treated with oral administration of sulfa medication. This would have to be acquired through the visit to a veterinary clinic unfortunately. Here the animal would probably show definite symptoms of not feeling up to par. The more watery the feces, the more potentially serious the problem could be especially if the pup shows secondary symptoms. If it piles up to any degree, I don't consider it diarrhea.

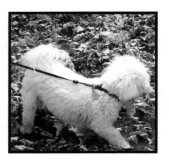

Notes

_____
_____
_____
_____
_____
_____
_____
_____
_____
_____
_____
_____
_____
_____
_____
_____
_____
_____
_____
_____
_____
_____
_____
_____

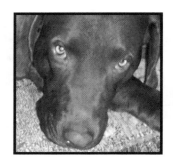# Chapter 6

VACCINATING FOR CORONA VIRUS

Vaccinating for corona virus is one of the sorriest jokes, I feel, that I have ever encountered. The American Animal Hospital Association goes so far as to say the disease doesn't exist. I've read that there has never been a recorded case in a dog past 8 weeks of age and I question whether there was ever anything of note in any dog younger. It's reported that the company that first patented the vaccine couldn't test if it worked because they weren't able to produce the disease in adult dogs. A veterinary salesman once confided in me that a researcher had told him he felt it was the best disease the salesman's company ever invented. I personally know several clinics that recommend it yearly. Here is another example, in my opinion, of unethical veterinarians wasting the client's money for personal gain and there is a lot of this vaccine sold nation wide!!! If they will mislead you on corona virus, what else will they deceive you on? DON'T VACCINATE FOR THIS!

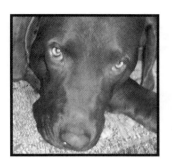

Notes

_____

_____

_____

_____

_____

_____

_____

_____

_____

_____

_____

_____

_____

_____

_____

_____

_____

_____

_____

_____

_____

_____

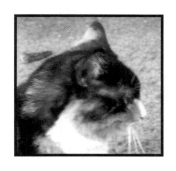

Chapter 7

KEEPING ELECTIVE SURGERY PATIENTS OVERNIGHT & PAIN MEDICATION

When you have simple elective surgery performed on your dog or cat and the clinic insists on keeping it overnight in order to more carefully monitor its recovery, is this a good idea? Not if they are charging you for the service and even if they don't, the animal will get closer monitoring at home and feel a lot more comfortable in the bargain. Here's why: Almost all veterinary establishments operate like any other business. They lock the door at five or six, go home and return at seven or eight the next morning. This means your animal is left totally unattended for over 12 hours. And you are charged for this? Wouldn't you rather have your pet home where it felt comfortable and where someone was actually looking after it?

Another area of ALMOST always unnecessary expense is pain medication following elective surgery. Before you think I'm an ogre, remember I'm speaking from a position of 25 or 30 thousand spays, neuters and declaws. I don't care what anyone says, animals recover much faster than people and with much less discomfort. In the first place a little soreness is nature's way of keeping the animal from being overactive after some injury. You can't tell them to take it easy. They do what they feel like. I have always sent my surgeries home the same day as the operation. Neuters are almost 100% normal at that time, spays are usually that way by evening and declaws only get into trouble if they are too active.

Do not pay for expensive pain medication. If you feel the animal needs some pain relief, give it simple aspirin at a rate of one 325 mg. tablet for each 50 to 60 lbs. of body weight twice daily. Cats are given the same weight dose only every 36 to 48 hours. Tylenol can be given at that same dose to dogs every 8 to 12 hours, but is NOT recommended for cats. People are primed to expect pain medication following surgery and rightfully so. But if the surgery is done right and stitched right, the animal will tolerate and often instigate hard play 24 hours later. I would wager this is something you wouldn't do so soon after a hysterectomy but dogs do. If your animal needs pain medication more than 24 hours after surgery, they must have used a chain saw to make the incision.

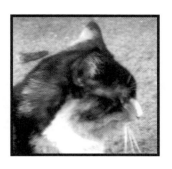

Notes

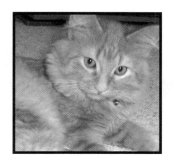

Chapter 8

DEMANDING HEALTH CHECKS & BLOOD TESTS BEFORE REFILLING PRESCRIPTIONS

This is another area of great abuse. Pet medical costs are a luxury and, in the vast majority of cases, simply can't take precedence over fixed living expenses for the average person. Veterinarians require frequent office visits on the pretense of needing to examine your pet before refilling its prescription. Often included in this is the drawing of blood in order to do a more thorough evaluation and the mandatory office call/exam fee. This is not exactly neither painless for your animal nor inexpensive. Your personal doctor will often give you a prescription with multiple refills but not your veterinarian.

Veterinarians make it an either or situation. You comply or else. Is it fair that your animal be forced to go without medication for a disease problem if you refuse to have tests ran? Shouldn't it be your decision to not run the tests? There is a risk with taking aspirin or Tylenol for God's sake yet you don't get tested before purchasing another bottle. You are the best placed person to judge any irregularities that might occur in the animal's general behavior. Granted there are some drugs that might be dangerous if not monitored, but not the vast majority of every day prescribed drugs and even then the risk is almost always slight. I do not think it is ethical to deny your pet its medication if you refuse the test. Veterinarians will almost always let your pet go WITHOUT medication if you refuse to let them extract $50 or more from you with a periodic exam between refills. This should be your decision after getting an HONEST appraisal of the risks without unjustified scare tactics. Examples of some products, that I feel are abused in this manner are: Pain medication, thyroid, phenobarbital for seizures, heartworm medication, urinary incontinence medication, wormers, and flea and tick prevention just to name just a few. You are at the mercy of the veterinarian here but, if you can't afford the cost of repeated tests before each prescription refill, try to find someone who is more reasonable and caring. Someone who would rather see your animal stays healthy by remaining on the medication rather than suffer a relapse without it. Complications with the medication SHOULD always be the lesser risk or it shouldn't be prescribed.

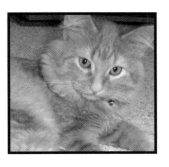

Notes

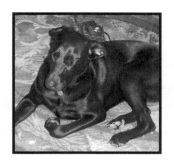

Chapter 9

ANNUAL TEETH CLEANING

Dentistry has been a godsend to the veterinary profession, as far as a generator of business and income is concerned. The profession implies that animals are no different than humans and need to be treated the same in regard with their teeth. If you believe this, I have a gold mine in Minnesota I will sell cheap. Animals have a lifespan a fraction that of humans, they do very little public speaking where a perfect smile is a necessity, they seldom chew their food before swallowing (probably the main reason they have bad teeth) and they couldn't care less about the condition of their teeth or whether they even have any. Yet twice a year dental checks are what most clinics shoot for. Money, money!

This is an area where there will be a lot of contention. I am speaking from a position of 40 years experience having had thousands of animals on my exam table with the vast majority declining any tooth work. I have not personally felt that lack of dental care had any serious effect on the life of the animal except the few very worst cases and I have seen some doozies. In the extremely bad cases, the dog's breath was so horrendous from rotten teeth that it was difficult to stand near it. It seemed to bother me more than the owners or the dog. Dentistry pushing veterinarians will imply that plaque and the resulting gum irritation are a real health threat to your pet. They can even state this will affect the animal's heart. Since I almost never see animals with diagnosable heart disease, I would strongly question this! The few heart problems I've seen usually have had pretty good teeth. I really doubt if the threat of premature death from the problem in the VAST majority of animals is any greater than that from the risk of repeatedly putting them under anesthesia for cleaning purposes. And then there is the cost of each visit. Putting older pets under anesthesia includes extensive presurgical screening which greatly adds to the expense of the procedure. I contend that it is simply not cost effective. I strongly feel the bulk of the tooth cleaning and oral surgery done today is mainly a generator of clinic income with minimal benefit to the animal.

Any chipped or broken tooth will automatically lead to the recommendation of a root canal for $500. I have NEVER seen a broken tooth bother a dog and I've seen hundreds. DON'T WASTE YOUR MONEY ON A ROOT CANAL! And don't spend a dime on tooth care in animals less than six months of age. Retained baby teeth will NOT damage the animal. They will catch a little more food but can be left if cost of removal is prohibitive. I have never known a retained baby tooth to create a problem that bothered the dog. The implication that they will push the permanent tooth out of alignment is almost never true and even if it was, wouldn't make the dog one iota of difference. Feeding a piece of raw chicken with bone intact would solve any problem of food buildup between the baby tooth and its neighbor and would keep the rest of the teeth in tip top shape also. (Feeding raw chicken explained below). I would highly recommend it twice a week. Brushing would also be an option.

Since large dogs have considerably less plaque build up and tooth problems than small dogs, it should be considered unethical to even suggest yearly dental exams on them. Generally, the smaller the dog, the greater the potential problems. Extreme cases in older, small dogs will cause many teeth to loosen and eventually fall out. These are times where cleaning solid teeth and extracting loose ones possibly justifies the cost. Of course limited feeding and brushing daily would have probably prevented the problem but few people have the intestinal fortitude to do this and many pets will not allow it. If you do brush, any toothpaste not toxic to you will be OK for your pet and anybody who tells you differently is trying to sell you something. Brushing just the outside of the teeth is all that's important. The inside stays pretty clean.

Another area to get gouged is in tooth extraction during a cleaning procedure. It's not unusual to see $50 added to the bill for each tooth pulled. The inside scoop is that a loose tooth pulls so easily it takes no more effort to remove it than it does to clean off the plaque. This is another way to pad the bill.

I have a client with a LARGE dog with an unusual (for a large breed dog) reoccurring plaque problem and she solved it by twice weekly giving it a WHOLE RAW chicken (it's a St Bernard). The toughness of the raw meat and crunching of the bones did an excellent job of cleaning its teeth. Nothing over the counter seems to do this. Pound per pound, this is probably as cheap as most moist dog foods and much better quality protein. A section of raw chicken wing (with meat attached) would be a good alternative for small dogs. An even better one for real small animals might be raw chicken necks. Chicken quarters can often be purchased very economically (Walmart) and would be good for slightly bigger animals. Raw bones are NOT a danger. Cooking hardens chicken bones and makes them more threatening. The attached meat requires a lot more chewing and pads the bone when it's swallowed. It may sound repulsive, but TRY it. Don't cut it up into small pieces. The requirement of chewing and tearing it into edible pieces is where the benefit arises. This actually makes a dog's teeth perform the function that nature and evolution intended. Do it on a regular basis, preferably twice a week. You can remove the skin and excess fat if fewer calories are desired. It can be fed frozen or thawed. Frozen would give the most benefit. It could save you a LOT in dental expenses and be much more pleasurable to the animal.

Pets don't like dental visits any more than you do and don't forget the anesthetic risk which is a much greater threat to your pet's life than any raw bone could ever be. Wild carnivores live on raw meat. If your dog won't eat raw, blanch and salt the outside just enough to add flavor but not enough to take away the toughness. You don't want to cook it. This method would be a LOT easier than brushing and probably much more effective. Milk bones are just dry dog food in another shape. They add calories to already over weight pets and don't clean the teeth. Most dental work can be declined with a very minimal effect on your pet and a great affect on savings. You can probably TOTALLY eliminate the need, by following the advice given above. If the animal's teeth are already falling out, it's probably a little late to expect miracles.

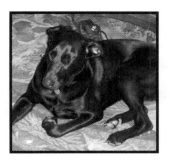

Notes

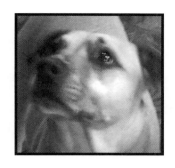

Chapter 10

X-RAYING EVERY LIMPING DOG

People are paranoid when it comes to their pet. Any animal that suddenly limps will often result in immediately rushing it to the doctor. Here is where common sense gets thrown out with the wash water. NO ANIMAL IS GOING TO DIE FROM A LIMP! Even an actual broken bone is not going to be fatal. Remember, animals can and do sprain their legs just as you do and most limps are of this nature. Almost all sprains will resolve themselves in a few days in spite of what you do. A severe injury elicits real (not imagined) pain. Even with a broken leg, rushing in after hours to an emergency clinic will only result in a greatly increased bill, without anything but emotional benefit to the owner, because almost never will work be performed before the following day. The animal will be medicated, put in a cage as soon as you leave and almost certainly not attended to, until the necessary personnel arrive during the next working day.

This may seem like very callus advice but remember this: IF YOU CAN'T AFFORD TO SPEND SEVERAL THOUSAND DOLLARS FIXING A POTENTIAL BROKEN LEG OR TORN JOINT LIGAMENT, DON'T GO IN AT ALL. AN X-RAY IS A WORTHLESS EXPENSE UNLESS YOU ARE WILLING TO PURSUE THE SURGICAL CORRECTION THAT IT MIGHT REVEAL. These surgical procedures cost thousands. Don't pay for an X-ray if you can't afford the surgery that follows. Ask questions first – not later. Anything not broken is very likely going to heal anyway and won't benefit from the x-ray.

If the animal steps on the foot at all, that's the best clue you have that nothing is broken. I repeat; dogs and cats are not going to die from a sore leg. Aspirin given at a rate of one 325mg. tablet for 50 to 60 lbs. of animal, twice daily for dogs and once every 48 hours for cats, is a good pain reliever. If you do take your animal in for examination of a limp, be forewarned that almost all clinics and hospitals will immediately recommend an X-ray. This generates income.

Even though most cases can be diagnosed with a simple exam, there's more money in the X-ray route. A broken leg will cost almost always in excess of several thousand dollars to fix. Again, if you can't afford that much or simply don't want to spend that much, don't waste your money on the X-ray!!! A lot of broken legs can heal so if your pet has the misfortune of this happening and you cannot afford surgical treatment, give it time. Above all, don't be talked into either expensive treatment if it's unaffordable or destroying the animal. If the worst case scenario happens and you end up with a dog with a chronic leg problem, keep its weight down, use inexpensive pain medication only when necessary (aspirin or Tylenol) and possibly a prednisone tablet every other day if you can find a veterinarian that is smart enough to use them. You would be surprised how well animals can get around on three legs. I've even known a couple that lived full lives with only two legs on one side.

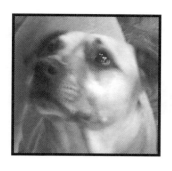

Notes

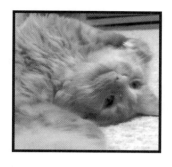

Chapter 11

PRESURGICAL SCREENING TESTS BEFORE ELECTIVE SURGERY

Presurgical screening constitutes drawing blood to run a CBC (complete blood count) and organ evaluation tests before surgery. It may also involve X-rays and heart evaluation. This of course greatly inflates the overall cost. The reason it's pushed and even insisted on is because it's done in human medicine and IT GENERATES INCOME. Litigation is the implied reason. The difference is that human doctors must be defensive of lawsuits. The risk of lawsuits in veterinary medicine are about 1/1000th that of doctors in the human field. The question is; is it necessary and worth the cost or just another way to produce more income for the clinic? Be forewarned that as animals acquire more rights in court, these tests will become mandatory whether they benefit the pet or not. California and animal rights activists are leading the way on pet's rights and they are probably going to push pet care costs out of sight.

Having personally had close to 30,000 dogs and cats under anesthesia in the past 40 years and having never lost one from anesthetic that presurgical screening would have prevented, I would say emphatically, NO! I have never had an animal presurgical screened in my life. The danger in anesthesia, and that is the biggest danger your pet will experience from routine operations, is directly related to the anesthetic used and the skill and experience of the doctor in charge. Sadly, many routine spay and neuter procedures are delegated to the newly hired graduate, who also has the least amount of experience. No amount of presurgical screening is going to compensate for lack of experience or expertise. It is just not cost effective in my experience, but presurgical screening is the wave of the future. If $100 had been spent presurgically screening every surgery I have performed, in the neighborhood of three million dollars would have been spent. Even if it would have saved one animal, I wouldn't call that cost effective.

Does presurgical screening really make a big difference? Consider this; I have never had an anesthetic fatality in any of the 15,000 dogs and cats I've spayed in my 40 years in practice. I know for a fact that a multiple doctor clinic I'm familiar with lost both a young dog and also a cat spay in the near past and that another large clinic in a nearby town also lost a cat spay during that same period. Both veterinary establishments insist on presurgical screening. I very strongly feel it is pushed only for the fact that it's mandatory in human medicine and it's another generator of income. If not done on a person and a problem occurred, the courts could hold the doctor liable, because all means had not been utilized to prevent any possibility of problems. The fact that the mishap probably occurred because the doctor was careless or inexperienced is usually not a consideration in court. You can be a bumbling idiot, but as long as all the tests are run, you will probably be exonerated.

I have known veterinarians, who insisted on running the gauntlet of tests before performing surgery in an emergency situation, as with a c-section, pulling porcupine quills or correcting a severe injury. If the tests showed that the animal wasn't in the best of shape, do you suppose they were going to wait a week or two before tending to the problem? I think tests demanded in these cases are absolutely stupid! The problem has to be addressed and it has to be done now! Here is where experience is worth its weight in gold in the handling of the anesthetic.

Have I ever had an anesthetic fatality? I have had several. There is one class of dogs (adult, unneutered, large breed male) that for some reason are at much greater risk when given intravenous anesthetics. This was something never mentioned in veterinary school, probably because they weren't aware of it. If the drug atropine is given 10 minutes before the anesthetic, the problem seems to be prevented. I had to acquire this piece of information by talking directly to the manufacturer of an anesthetic. This fact was not included on the information sheet that accompanied the bottle of drug. I honestly feel that, if I had been privy to this knowledge 25 years ago, I would never have lost a dog. Why the company was so reluctant to share this information, I will never know. Presurgical screening would never have prevented these anesthetic fatalities. Here again, experience is worth much more and doesn't result in a big added on fee that isn't justifiable in my experience.

Find an older veterinarian who does all the surgery himself, who comes with good recommendations and save the cost of presurgical screening. Be forewarned that office staffs are often coached to approach you in relays trying to talk you into the presurgical screening. It's a money maker and they will try to imply you are risking your pet's life if it isn't done. Find an older vet with a lot of experience and forego the testing on routine surgeries. I feel you will be better off. That way you will NOT be paying extra to prevent a problem that would much more likely be a result of the doctor's ineptitude rather than due to a weakness with the animal's system. I feel an experienced veterinarian with a sound record and just doing the surgery would be a much better investment than a newer graduate doing the operating and charging you for the tests.

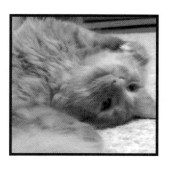

Notes

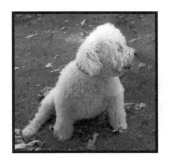

Chapter 12

YEAR AROUND HEARTWORM PREVENTION

Quite simply, if there are no mosquitoes, your pet can't get heartworm. And mosquitoes are not instantly infectious. Under ideal conditions, it takes two weeks for a mosquito to be dangerous after biting an infected dog. Ideal conditions require the temperature to remain consistently above 70 degrees. Periodic dips below 70 degrees greatly slow development of the parasite in the mosquito. Since the preventive will eliminate any exposure for the previous 45 days, it is hard to justify starting treatment sooner than 2 months after the appearance of mosquitoes.

This is the advice I gave in the seasonal climate in which I live. Many veterinarians imply that year around prevention makes the pet owner less apt to forget. What do you think? I think they are just trying to sell you more preventative. There is also the fact that some heartworm preventatives contain a second ingredient (which you pay extra for) that helps treat and prevent intestinal worms. They are forcing you to worm your dog every month, whether you want to or not. Treating for intestinal parasites several times a year is often a good idea but monthly is probably overkill, except for large groups of animals raised in close confinement. If you feel that monthly worming for intestinal parasites is a good idea, purchase bulk wormer (explained in worming chapter 28) and don't waste your money on unnecessary heart worm medication.

Is year around prevention necessary? If it's too cold for mosquitoes, you can't get heartworm. In fact, according to the American Heartworm Society, if the temperature isn't consistently above 70 degrees, the parasite won't mature in a mosquito. Alaska has a jillion mosquitoes but no heartworm. The temperature is too cool to develop in the insects. If you live in Florida, year around prevention is a good idea. If you live in northern Minnesota, treating from the end of June through October is probably all you need.

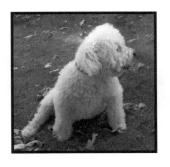

Notes

_____

_____

_____

_____

_____

_____

_____

_____

_____

_____

_____

_____

_____

_____

_____

_____

_____

_____

_____

_____

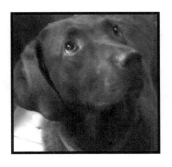

Chapter 13

YEAR AROUND FLEA & TICK PREVENTION

Flea and tick preventives are also strongly overused. Flea threat ranges from year around in southern climates to only a few months in the northern U.S. If it's freezing, there will be no fleas outside. They like warm and moist. The only way your pet will contact them in cold weather is directly from an infected animal that is visiting your home or from your visit to a home with a problem. So treating when there isn't a threat is not a good investment in my mind.

Ticks are more durable and some show up with the spring thaw and remain until hard freezes in the fall. This is especially true of the deer ticks which have the most potential for carrying diseases.

The need to use preventive varies from the absolute paranoid who can't stand the thought of one on their precious pet to someone who couldn't care less if the animal was covered and I've seen a number of these. If you are willing to pick an occasional tick and your animal only gets a few, it's hard to justify $12 to $15 a month preventive costs. If you live on a lake and the dog swims every day, it's probably a waste of money also. I've lived in tick country all my life and I have never seen a tick bite become infected on a dog. People yes—dogs no. A little swelling on a dog will be gone in a week or so. The head does NOT get buried.

For those who treat their animals in order to prevent the ticks from being brought into the house to threaten the owner, you're probably deluding yourselves. The preventatives only potentially kill the tick if it's attached to the dog or trying to attach. It probably has very little effect on ticks that are just crawling in and on the fur looking for a spot to burrow in. These are the ones that can shed off and possibly choose you for their meal. I don't honestly think treating the animal will lessen your chance of getting a tick this way.

I don't personally feel any of the pet store products are effective enough to warrant bringing home for either fleas or ticks. The main veterinary ones are Frontline Plus, Advantix and Revolution. None are 100% but do prevent most ticks. I like Frontline the best because it can be used on both cats and dogs. If you have a confirmed case of fleas, ALL the animals in the household need to be treated to correct the problem.

A MONEY SAVING TIP: Frontline and the other two mentioned products come in usually four different sizes to treat a specific weight of dog. The cost for each size is about the same. You will be sold three or six small vials of the product specific for your dog's weight to put on the animal's back at monthly intervals. Each size will treat two dogs of the NEXT SMALLER size. If you have a small dog, you can buy a bigger size, get multiple treatments from it and greatly lower your cost. The manufacturers have for seen this possibility and consequently put their products in containers that are impossible to measure part doses out of for smaller animals. (Nice people)! You will need an empty syringe to draw the vial contents into to accurately distribute it on the dog. The largest dog size of Frontline Plus holds 4 ml (cc) of liquid and this will treat an 89 to 130 lb. dog. Thus 1 ml would treat a 25 to 30 lb. dog (4 treatments for the price of one). If you think you can handle this, it will result in a savings. The stuff is quite non toxic if you accidentally overdose it. ¼ of a teaspoon will hold enough Frontline to treat a 30 to 35 lb. dog. Preferably obtain a 5 or 6 cc or ml syringe, transfer the contents into the syringe and apply the measured amount directly from the syringe ONTO THE ANIMAL'S BACK.

You should be able to obtain a 3cc and a 6cc syringe from a farm store that sells large animal vaccines or over the internet. Get also several 18 or 20 gauge needles one inch or 1½ inches long. Snap the top of the vial to let in air. Put a needle on the larger syringe, pierce the bottom corner of the vial with the needle and draw all of the contents into the syringe. Then you can use the 3cc syringe to measure doses to administer onto the animal. NO NEEDLE ON THIS SYRINGE. Pull the plunger to the desired dose (1/2 cc for 13 lbs., 1cc for 25 lbs., 1 1/3 cc for 35 lbs. etc.), stick the needle of the full syringe in the open end of the smaller syringe and gently fill the 3cc syringe to the tip. Then carefully squirt the dose ON the animal's skin between the shoulder blades. REMEMBER YOU ARE NOT INJECTING. Repeat the procedure for other animals at whatever dose is needed. Don't forget cc and ml is the same. Administer at a dose of 1cc for each 25 or 30 pounds of dog or cat. The dog Frontline can be used on a cat and one large sized (89 to 132 lb.) dose will treat 8 or 10 adult cats very economically. Any veterinarian who tells you this can't be done is trying to sell you something!

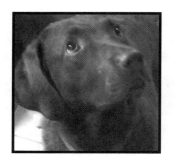

Notes

_____

_____

_____

_____

_____

_____

_____

_____

_____

_____

_____

_____

_____

_____

_____

_____

_____

_____

_____

_____

_____

_____

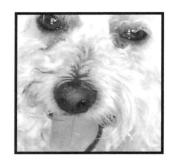

Chapter 14

WELLNESS EXAMS ONCE OR TWICE YEARLY

This sounds like a good, health promoting idea but think about how often you get a check up from your doctor. I feel that this is a blatant ploy to get you in the door to extract money on a biannual basis. I even read recently that not everyone in the medical field was convinced that annual human checkups were worth the time and expense. Personally I feel that you are as good a judge of your pet's general well being as anyone. Good rule of thumb: if you feel your pet isn't acting up to par and the condition lasts long enough to be a concern, then have it checked out. Twice a year check ups on normal animals are in my opinion another way to get the client in the door on a more frequent basis to "make work" without real benefit to the animal. My recommendation would be to schedule checkups when you think it's necessary, if at all.

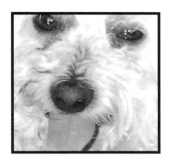

Notes

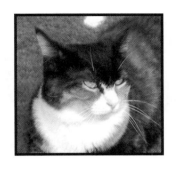 # Chapter 15

RECOMMENDING EXPENSIVE SURGERY WITHOUT OFFERING LESS COSTLY OPTIONS

Don't rush into elective surgery. A lot of things will heal if you give them a little time. Some things take weeks. A non growing limp is not going to kill an animal. If money is tight, just keeping the animal's weight down will allow it to function very well even when favoring a leg. I read a report from one of the veterinary schools where they did NOT advocate surgery for hip dysplasia. They very strongly felt that keeping the animal's weight down, walking and swimming for exercise rather than running and an inexpensive 5 mg. prednisone tablet every other day resulted in as good a life for the dog as thousands of dollars worth of surgery. If surgery is recommended, get a second opinion from some veterinarian who is not "knife happy", if you can find one. Look at the dog and think about how it affects the animal's behavior. Often you are treating your emotions more than the perceived pain of the animal. Never do hip displasia surgery on a dog under a year of age because it is very difficult to positively diagnose it that young and you would in all probability be operating for no valid reason.

As an example of knife happy doctors and not getting a second opinion, consider this true, personal story: About 15 years ago an orthopedic surgeon wanted to do a bilateral shoulder joint replacement on my wife. At that time a shoulder joint replacement had a life span of 3 to 5 years and then had to be redone. Fortunately I was a veterinarian with medical training and common sense. We declined this advice of a specialist! I am a big believer in healthy eating, vitamins at much higher than FDA recommendations, supplements and exercise. She did her own self imposed physical therapy so she wouldn't lose range of movement. We both got on glucoseamine/chondroitin (explained in arthritis section) shortly thereafter and her shoulders are basically normal today. That doctor would have ruined her life. I don't like to think how many painful and unnecessary human joint surgeries are performed every year. If people were willing to change their diet and life style, there is often a much better alternative. But remember that non surgical alternatives are not suggested, because the MONEY IS IN THE SURGERY.

IMPLYING PROCEDURES
THAT HAVE TO BE DONE

When a veterinarian says something has to be done, consider changing doctors. No veterinarian is a policeman, so no one has given him/her the right to be an enforcer of some imaginary law.

The only thing that has to be done is to vaccinate for rabies in order to cross borders, get a pet license for the animal, or operate a day or foster care center. Boarding kennels demand vaccinations in order to keep your animal and they will probably demand they be done oftener than necessary. If you need them for boarding, you will have to comply. It's your pet and it should always be your choice.

ALWAYS ask the reason for the recommended procedure and demand detail why it's necessary and what the benefit will be. Most demanded procedures are in the make work category. And almost all will result in follow up care that can cost big bucks. Ask first what the procedure will accomplish and the following costs. Be forewarned that almost all veterinary clinics will DEMAND the pet be vaccinated when you bring it in the door. There is NO valid justification for this except a profit motive. It takes probably a week for a vaccination to impart protection to a previously unvaccinated animal.

Your personal doctor will strongly recommend your children receive early childhood inoculations but most assuredly will NOT refuse to treat them if you decline. Your children will live many decades longer than your pet but the vaccinations will almost certainly never be repeated. Most veterinarians will demand they be repeated multiple times and refuse to treat them if you don't. What does this tell you about their ethics and profit motive?

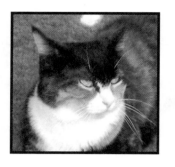

Notes

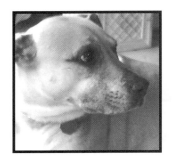

Chapter 16

CHECKING THE ANIMAL'S TITER

A titer is supposedly the level of antibodies an animal has in its blood stream as a result of exposure to the actual disease or from a vaccination. Theoretically the higher the titer, the more protection an animal has against that certain disease causing organism.

Checking an animal's titer is a new wrinkle in order to make up for drop in income due to decreased vaccination frequency. The veterinarian will imply that it is necessary to be sure your dear animal is really protected. Remember this will result in sticking a needle in the dog's front leg to draw blood. The AVMA has stated that in theory it's a good idea but in actuality, it probably has no bearing on an animal's actual protection. Animals with no discernable titer have been found to be as resistant to disease exposure as those with titers that register fairly high. If your animal has been vaccinated any time after 6 months of age— DON'T WASTE YOUR MONEY! Another ploy to get you in the door on a yearly basis is staggering the vaccinations. Ever since vaccinations have been given, combining them all together has been the norm and still is in humans, but now you may be told it's best to separate them and give a different one yearly. Don't be fooled.

I just came across, what appears in my mind, to be a new, devious method to extract more money from a client while still appearing to be a concerned doctor. A clinic came up with the idea where a titer check is ran to see if "Fluffy" is protected. The charge is $40. If the titer "appears" to be low, a "free" vaccination is given.

Analysis:
a. A mature animal who has been vaccinated doesn't need a booster.
b. The titer check has been deemed virtually worthless.
c. You spend $40 with only the clinic benefiting.
d. An uninformed client thinks he/she has a caring veterinarian. Smart!!

I was just reading where Leptospirosis vaccinations are now being recommended yearly (they can't get away from that yearly thing) along with kennel cough yearly or even TWICE yearly. In 40 years I have never seen a case of what I felt was either Lepto or kennel cough. The latter is a contagious bronchitis that would result in a deep cough lasting a week or so but would probably resolve itself much like flu cough would if you had it. I see a lot of bronchitis cases (coughing) but they've responded to simple antibiotics, meaning they were probably of bacterial origin and not viral.

They have never been a serious problem. The dog usually never even acted sick and it seldom has spread to other animals. Why such a big deal is made over it I have never understood. Nor have I ever encountered a case of Lepto which is a bacteria possibly affecting the kidneys. I don't vaccinate my dogs for either of these and I have never recommended my clients do so either, even though I could have probably increased my income substantially by doing so. I am sure many veterinarians can hype them up to be absolutely necessary. I would personally not be worried about either one. If you do choose to vaccinate, repeating yearly in my opinion is another "make work" scam.

Once an animal has been programmed to produce immunity from the stimulation of a vaccine, it lasts many, many years. Why would these vaccines need to be repeated any more often then once or twice during the life of the pet???? I feel it's just another way to get you in the door and generate extra income. If your dog develops a mild cough and your veterinarian chastises you for not vaccinating for kennel cough, remember this-----unless the good doctor has valid laboratory conformation as to the exact cause, he/she has no clue as to the causative organism. There are dozens of things out there that can make you or your animal cough.

I recently read that the Lepto vaccination usually doesn't even contain the right strains of the Leptospiral organism that would be expected to affect a dog. How's that for wasting your money and risking the animal's health?

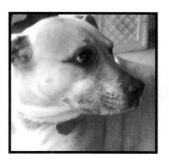

Notes

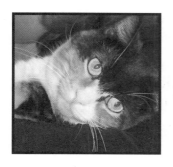

Chapter 17

SURGICAL REMOVAL OF EVERY SMALL LUMP OR BUMP

A couple stopped in one time for a second opinion on an old lab with a small, quarter sized lump in one flank. Another veterinarian from the Twin Cities had seized on this and implied it was definitely a cancer. He recommended immediate removal. Of course an old dog would require extensive testing before the surgery and he was even preparing them for chemotherapy following the removal. I told them it looked like a thousand other lumps I've seen in geriatric dogs over the years and not to worry about it. If and ONLY if it started to enlarge dramatically, then consider having it removed. Based on many years experience, I did not expect that to happen. Even with removal, the chemo therapy ploy was a joke with this type of lump.

Old dogs get a lot of small cysts, fatty tumors, warts and lumps found on, in and under the skin. Fortunately almost all of these are of no consequence to the pet's health. If it's small (quarter sized or so), not growing and not bothering the animal, don't let anyone make an expense out of it. Threatening tumors are VERY rare and grow steadily. The majority of the ones I have seen were involving bone or were mammary tumors. Most large, soft masses on older dogs are fatty tumors which are NOT a threat and need to be removed only if they interfere with movement. Warts on top of the skin are common in old dogs and are removed only for cosmetic reasons or if the animal scratches them and makes them bleed. They won't hurt the animal. A biopsy may be recommended for a suspicious growth, but the total cost of that probably wouldn't be much less than simple removal without the biopsy and I would recommend the latter. Unspayed, older dogs are very likely to develop mammary tumors and these can be dangerous. I've almost never seen one on a spayed dog. Chemotherapy is expensive and, if it's really necessary, will probably only prolong the pet's life for a year. Ask questions in detail before proceeding.

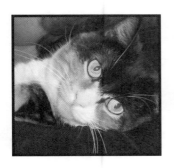

Notes

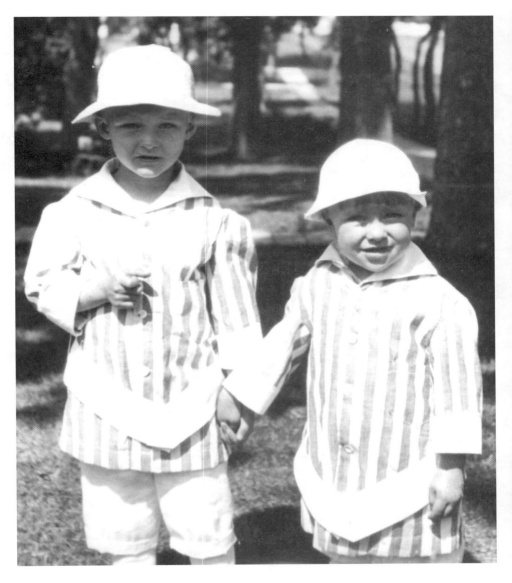

Father on left and Uncle on right. Both will become future veterinarians. Photo token in early 1920s.

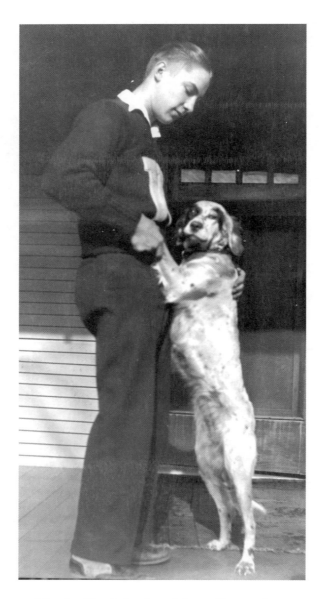

Uncle Bud during his college days
around 1940.

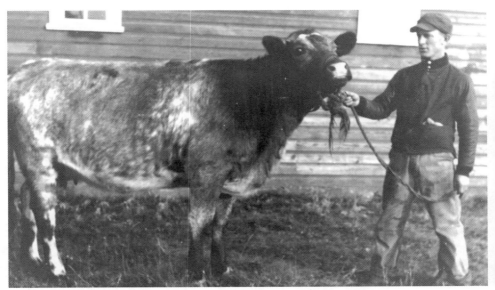

My grandfather who wasn't a veterinarian but fathered two boys
who would become veterinarians.

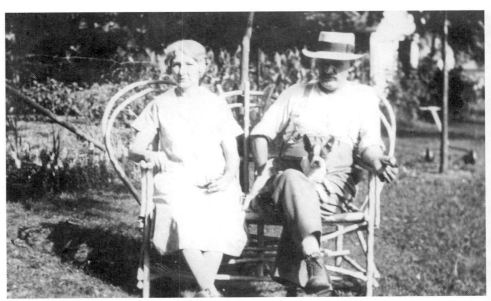

Dr. Krull and wife Kathryn. The original old "horse doctor"
who migrated to NE Nebraska from Michigan in the early
1900s. He had a thing for Boston terriers.

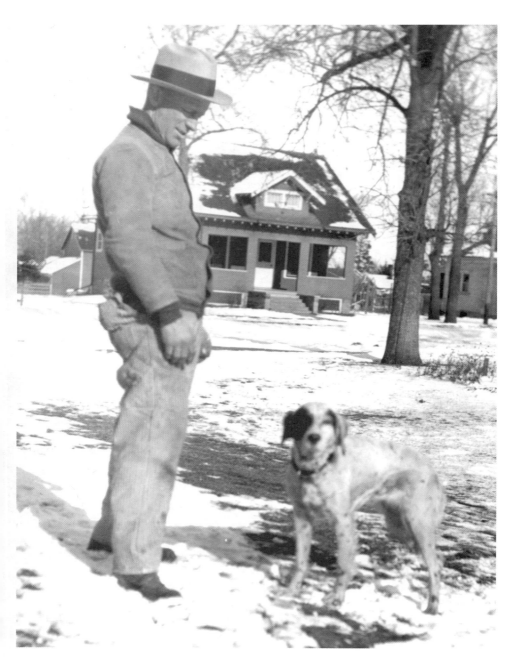

Grandfather Byron who was a postmaster.

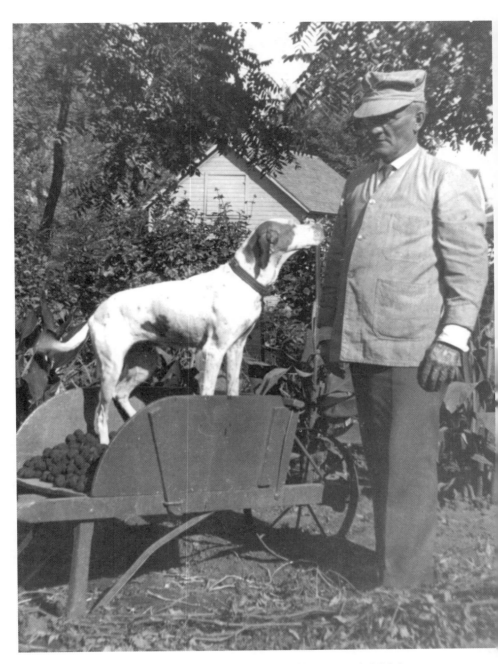

Great grandfather Dr. Krull around 1930

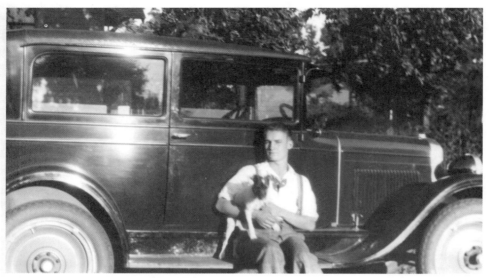

My father shortly after graduating in the mid 1930s

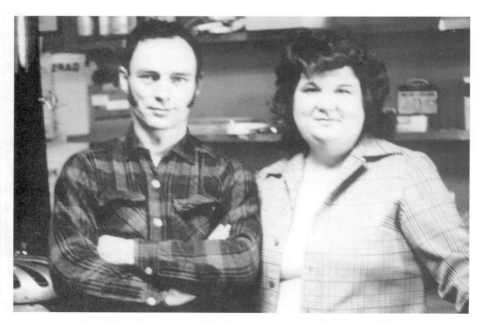

Dr. Busby and wife Marty in the late 1960s

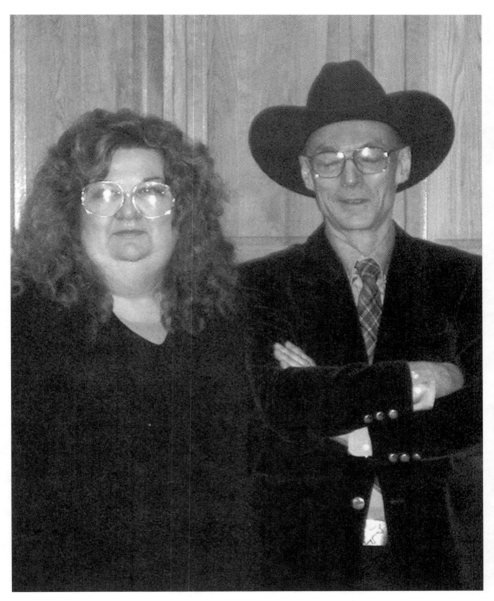

Dr. Busby and wife Marty in 2005. I blinked!

Part 2

Miscellaneous Advice

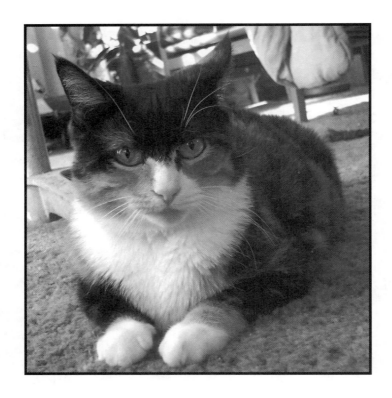

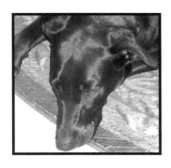

Chapter 18

OVER WEIGHT ANIMALS

Keep your animal's weight down. The majority of pets I have seen over the years were over weight. If it doesn't have a narrow waistline, it is probably too fat. This is the best health benefit you can give your pet and I read it may add one or two years more to the pet's life. KEEP IT LEAN. This will greatly reduce your need for veterinary care and save you enough money to enable you to afford what little care that might be required.

HOW MUCH TO FEED YOUR PET

If a dog weighs the right amount, you can feed it a little more during the active summer and fall seasons and then cut back during the winter when it tends to "couch potato" a lot more. If it's losing its waistline, you are feeding it too much and on the way to incurring a lot of otherwise unnecessary veterinary expenses.

AVOID VETERINARIANS WHO TRY TO SHAME YOU

If a veterinarian tries to shame you into accepting an expensive procedure or implies you are a derelict and uncaring owner to not treat your animal in the way he or she advises, GET A DIFFERENT VETERINARIAN.

I never knew my great grandfather, Dr. Krull. He passed on seven years before I was born. One naturally hears stories over the years about a relative like that and one came from a farmer I had as a client shortly after graduating veterinary school. The farmer was an older man by that time and recalled an incident where he and his father had called Dr. Krull out to treat a horse with colic. Colic is an all inclusive term for any gastro/intestinal upset a horse might encounter ranging all the way from mild indigestion to invariably fatal intestinal blockage. My grandfather had apparently arrived on the scene in his trusty Model T and drove up close to the pen where the patient was awaiting his arrival. As he parked the car, the farmer walked up to his side of the car and the two batted the breeze for several minutes. While carrying on the conversation, Dr. Krull was naturally observing the animal. After a few minutes passed he started the car and said he had to go. "Aren't you going to treat the horse" the farmer asked? All my grandfather said was "He'll die" and away he went. This was in a time where trip charges and mileage hadn't yet been invented. "Well, that wasn't good enough for us," the farmer related so they got another vet to come out from a town in the opposite direction. Upon his arrival and exam, this second veterinarian said he thought he could save the horse. "It died"! The farmer said. They never doubted him after that. What probably happened was that the horse must have vomited while my grandfather was watching. It is my understanding that with a horse showing colic, vomiting is a sure sign of total intestinal blockage and early 1920's you could kiss that one good bye. You probably could today too.

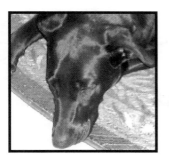

Notes

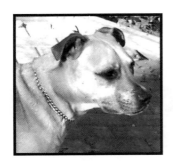

Chapter 19

ARTHRITIS (OSTERARTHRITIS) IN OLD DOGS

Large breed, old dogs almost always get osteoarthritis in the rear end when they reach or pass 10 years of age. Many veterinarians prescribe expensive daily pain pills. Don't forget aspirin or Tylenol may work. Some favor a product called Cosequin. This works well and is my favorite but you can save scads of money by getting the same thing at a local store. Don't let a veterinarian tell you these shouldn't be used on dogs.

Look for a generic product in the supplement/vitamin section for arthritis in any discount store that contains 500 mg. of glucoseamine and 400 mg. of chondroitin PER capsule. It shouldn't cost more than $20.00 per 100 capsules. Give at least one pill morning and night. It will be the same ingredients and cost a fraction. The first month I recommend giving two pills in the AM and one in the PM as a test. If no improvement is seen in a month, don't waste any more money on that treatment. If it works, and it usually does, maintain the animal on one capsule AM and one PM. This is a VERY effective treatment for osteoarthritis in people also and virtually side effect free. If you have a problem, try it the same way described above for a month and evaluate the results. If it's a benefit, stay on at least one capsule morning and evening. It will sure beat surgery. Remember there are three options for your dog: Pain pills (the expensive veterinary dispensed ones or aspirin and Tylenol), the inexpensive steroid prednisone (5 mg. daily or every other day) which most younger veterinarians hate but which some older veterinarians (me included) think are great, and glucoseamine/chondroitin given as described above. Most over the counter pain pills can probably be given with no more danger to the pet than there would be to you. Remember thousands of people suffer serious stomach bleeding and possible stomach perforations every year from taking these very same pain relievers and yet have no hesitation of using them. I doubt if your pet would be in any more danger and probably not as much. Just don't overdose it on a small animal. The prescribed veterinary pain pills probably carry just as much risk. If a vet clinic demands periodically testing your animal before refilling your prescription, they would be hard pressed to claim theirs was more risk free.

There is a lot of pro and con on giving over the counter pain pills to pets. Aspirin and Tylenol are the preferred ones but I have had MANY situations where clients said they gave any number of different types of these pain medications to their animals. I have never known a time where one had any trouble. Some would even give a 10 or 15 pound animal a whole tablet. This is obviously a terrible overdose that wouldn't be recommended but I've yet to experience any problem as a result. You can take my experience for what it's worth. Use only aspirin on cats.

I know veterinary practices that routinely test for Lyme disease if your dog comes in with a limp. I consider this a total waste of time and money (yours-not theirs).

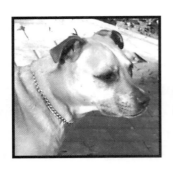

Notes

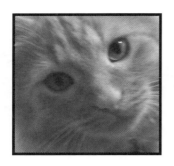

Chapter 20

TOOTHPASTE AND SHAMPOO

When you bathe your pet, any shampoo or soap you can use on yourself and your children will work equally as well on the animal. It's the same with brushing its teeth. Don't buy more expensive pet products. You can bathe a dog as often as necessary. Your hair doesn't dry up and fall out with repeated washings and neither will the dogs'. I've used hand soap, dish soap and any number of different shampoos---whatever was handy at the time. Even consider dandruff shampoo for dandruff.

VITAMINS FOR YOUR PET

Any vitamin product you take can also be given to your animal. Try to divide it somewhat according to the animal's weight when compared to yours.

WHAT PET FOOD IS BEST

There are dozens of different brands of pet foods on the market. Does it pay to feed only the higher priced brands? I personally doubt it. I once read where a nutritionist felt that the real expensive brands were probably no better than the older, middle priced ones that have been around for decades and have a reputation to uphold. These are what I feed my animals.

100

Veterinarians carry and push the elite and more expensive brands and make a profit when you purchase from them. They will also imply the brand they sell is the only one you should feed. Remember they can mislead about other things too when profit is involved.

I'm not pushing any brand but I feed my dogs and cats Gaines or Purina. I would recommend any reputable puppy chow for the first year and then any adult food after that. A real active dog might benefit from a higher protein but sometimes the protein source in cheaper dog foods comes from poor and possibly even indigestible sources. Most active dogs will do fine on any reputable adult food. Very few pets get enough physical activity to warrant real high protein dog food! Compared to a sled dog running many miles daily, your animal is probably a pansy. Old dogs move less and eat just as much so go to a lower calorie food like senior or even diet food for them and cut portion sizes. I have had dogs come in the clinic that just shined. When I would ask the owner what brand of food the animal was fed, the answer was never consistent. The brand named would range from one of the cheaper foods one time on up to an expensive one the next. You figure!

WHEN & HOW TO GIVE PETS A BITE OF FOOD

If you are smart (I've learned from experience) you won't give treats during your meal. Make them wait until your last spoonful and then offer a bite. It will make for a lot pleasanter dining time. Otherwise the pet will expect to share every other mouthful. Most importantly as far as keeping the pet's weight down, a small fingernail sized piece will be just as satisfying as the whole cookie.

OVER FEEDING YOUR PET

Excess weight on dogs and cats cause just as many health problems as in people. Keeping your animal lean could very easily result in its living one or two years longer. If it has lost its waistline, it is too heavy. You can almost NEVER feed as much as is recommended on the pet food container. They like to sell more and make money too. Each animal is different in its requirements and an active pet will require more just like active people do. Animals and people also vary with the seasons due to changes in activity levels in how many calories they need.

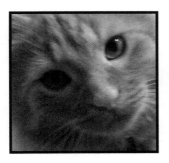

Notes

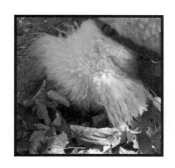

Chapter 21

CAT BITE INFECTIONS

Cats fight with other cats and sometimes develop an infection at the site of the bite. This is probably the most common reason for a sore leg in a cat. They will run a fever for several days. There will be a VERY tender and sore swelling at the site of the bite. Then an abscess will form and break open. A terrible looking wound will suddenly appear that looks absolutely gross but by this time the animal will probably have returned to normal activity. If you take it in to a veterinarian, all that needs to probably be done is to put it on simple antibiotics for a few days. DO NOT let them keep the animal and waste a lot of your money debriding the wound. I have seen hundreds in my life and some wounds were as large as a silver dollar. ALL healed up without a scar. I personally think the antibiotic is optional, if not given until after the abscess breaks open. By then the infection has progressed to the healing point. If the antibiotics are started soon enough, the abscess will not form and break open. Skip the tests and expensive cleaning. Just give antibiotics.

EAR INFECTIONS AND EAR MITES

External ear infections are common especially in hairy, long eared dogs. I would recommend treating with ear drops containing antibiotic, possibly a fungicide and preferably a steroid (cortisone) first. Oral antibiotics are not as effective. DO NOT let them talk you into leaving the animal for expensive ear flushing and sensitivity testing. Save those heroics for the few unresponsive cases. Try ear drops containing a broad spectrum antibiotic (gentamicin or baytril are excellent) combined with a steroid. Otomax or its generic equivalent has been my first choice. Ears DO NOT have to be cleaned before treating but common sense says it's probably a good idea. Why waste money running tests at first when something this simple is so effective. NO DOG IS GOING TO DIE FROM AN EAR INFECTION! Five drops of Otomax daily for 5 to 7 days are all that is needed. Very rarely does this not work. If that doesn't get the ear back to normal in a week, THEN consider clinic testing.

You can clean the animal's ear with the same cotton swab you use in your ears. Rubbing alcohol is what I use for cleaner on both normal and infected ears. It cuts the wax and doesn't seem to irritate even a raw, inflamed ear. Normal ears can be cleaned as seldom or as often as odor and wax build up dictate. You will NOT damage anything as long as the swab is vertical and you don't push unusually hard. The swab will descend about ½ to 1 inch until it hits the bottom of the ear. The ear drum is another ½ inch further in on a horizontal plain. It would be very difficult to damage it. Keep changing to new swabs until they come out fairly clean. Some dogs have more ear wax than others just like some people. Getting a dog up on a table top (like the exam table in a vet clinic), making it lay down and facing away from you will give you a tremendous advantage.

Swimming will not create a problem in the average dog. If you own an animal that has reoccurring ear infections, then drying the ears out with swabs immediately after swimming would probably pay dividends.

Cats and young puppies can have ear mites and adult dogs have ear infections. If there is a noticeable amount of black in cats' or puppies' ears, deep down, mites are almost always indicated. It will NOT hurt to treat for mites under these circumstances especially if the animal is itching its ear. Treat all the cats in your household at the same time or you won't get rid of the problem. Try treating for that first and if the problem persists, then check with your vet. Four to five drops of any mite medicine in each ear daily for five days should be sufficient.

Mites will not damage the ear. They just itch. No one dies from it and you can't catch this type of mite. Adult dogs can get ear mites but they seem much more resistant then when they were puppies. They get ear infections and this is confirmed by looking for redness. I have never seen redness and inflammation with mites. One ear is usually much more inflamed than the other. This needs to be treated with antibiotic drops—not oral pills. Simple cleaning with a swab first is all that's needed—don't get talked into letting them flush. ADULT DOGS GET INFECTIONS, ADULT CATS GET MITES AND PUPPIES AND KITTENS GET MITES. There are a few exceptions but not many. The black will persist in a cat's ear for a month or two following successful treatment. Don't worry about it as it will eventually disappear. If you treat an infected ear for mites, it won't hurt anything. It just won't get any better until you use antibiotics.

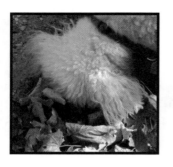

Notes

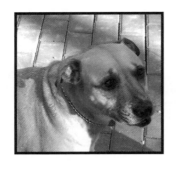

Chapter 22

CLIPPING NAILS AND TORN TOENAILS

Clipping a pet's nails can be challenging to a lot of people and intimidating besides.

Rule No. 1:

NO ANIMAL IS GOING TO BLEED TO DEATH FROM A NAIL CLIPPED TOO CLOSELY. But try not to do it too often because where there is blood there are also nerves and some degree of pain will be inflicted. Too many mistakes and your pet may run screaming under the bed when he sees you with the clippers.

Rule No. 2:

Restraint is crucial. It generally is best to have two people: a holder and a clipper. You will have the most control placing the animal on a slick counter or table top preferably narrow enough for someone to work from either side. The exam table in a veterinary clinic is a good example. Here is what you "attempt" to do: The holder faces the same direction as the pet. The arm closest to the animal goes over its back with the thumb up, the fingers down and the front of the hand forced into the animal's arm pit. This will enable you to keep it from backing up. You can keep the animal snuggled against your side and pressed on the table top this way. If it struggles, DON'T LET IT RISE UP-

--use your arm and body weight to gently but firmly press it flat on the table.

Your other hand goes UNDER the neck with the arm close to the pet's chest. Extend your reach far enough so your hand can literally grab a hand full of skin where the ear is attached. You heard me—grab a liberal hand full of skin on the far side of the head encompassing the whole ear in the process. It gives you something to grab on to and in the thousands of times I have done it there seems to be no pain to the animal. Massaging it when you aren't hanging on for dear life is comforting to the pet and rewards it for not fighting. If you maintain your grip, hold the head firmly against your chest and keep your arm tight against the animal's throat and chest, it can't bite you. I have seen a number of dogs throw a real fit when restrained for the first time but if you gently lay on it, hold the head firmly against you and don't let it get loose and win, they will accept defeat and give up. SOMEONE HAS TO BE BOSS AND YOU WILL BE A LOT HAPPIER IF IT ISN'T THE ANIMAL!!! If you think this is rough and cruel, how do you suppose the groomer or veterinary assistant do it?

Rule No.3:

How close to clip can be easy or difficult depending on a number of factors. White or light colored nails are easy. Look at the nail from the side and determine where the pink color (blood) ends and stay outside this a fifth of an inch or so. Dark nails make seeing the demarcation line between where the blood ends and where it's safe to clip impossible, so look at the underside and see if there is a hollow section toward the front. You can always cut the hollow part UP TO where the solid begins without getting into trouble. The solid black ones with no hollow underneath are a challenge. My suggestion is to guess at the right spot and to slowly squeeze the clipper without cutting. If you are too close to the quick, the animal will flinch noticeably. Moving far enough out won't elicit this pinching sensation and should be a safe place to cut. Trial and error and experience!

Rule No. 4:

If you hit blood, remember the world will not come to an immediate end. Here there are three choices to handle the problem: The first is to stop the bleeding with a styptic (silver nitrate) stick. This will cauterize the wound but cause more pain so it probably isn't a good choice. The second is to boot the animal outdoors for 20 minutes and let the blood clot normally as Mother Nature intended. The third is to gently snug a soft piece of cotton, Kleenex, gauze or whatever over the nail with a piece of tape and ignore it for an hour. This keeps it from getting blood all over the rugs and furniture. Hydrogen peroxide does a marvelous job getting blood out of fabric.

Rule No. 5:

Have someone else clip the nails. Cat nails are always white which makes where to clip easy to judge and they can always be clipped with a regular fingernail clipper. The challenge is in the restraint. On the table top just as with the dog gives you the best advantage. They can't be held the same but keeping them down on the surface and in the center of the table gives the best control. Holding them gently against your side with your other hand OVER the neck instead of under is effective. The more GENTLY they are held, the better. Constant massaging of the head and ears helps immensely.

When a dog tears a toenail, it usually results in a limp and a rush to the veterinarian. All that can be done is to clip off as much of the broken nail as possible so it doesn't touch the ground when the animal walks which creates pain. If money is tight, this is something that will almost always be self correcting in a week or so without doing anything but giving aspirin for as long as necessary. It's the same as if you tore your fingernail. Clip it as close as possible and give it time to heal. Only once or twice have I seen a toe become infected as a result. If pain persists and that toe becomes noticeably swollen compared to its neighbors, then oral antibiotics would be indicated.

If you encounter the unusual situation where a rear dew claw or deformed nail grows into such a tight circle that a regular clipper won't fit over it, a side cutter used for cutting wire will work well. Rarely a nail will curl and actually grow right into the flesh. Just clip it off in the middle and the wound should heal uneventfully.

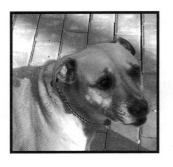

Notes

_____
_____
_____
_____
_____
_____
_____
_____
_____
_____
_____
_____
_____
_____
_____
_____
_____
_____
_____
_____
_____
_____
_____
_____

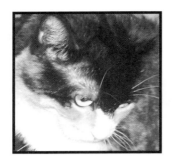# **Chapter 23**

CATARACTS AND LOSS OF HEARING

Virtually all old dogs develop cataracts and hearing loss if they live long enough. The cataracts appear as a gradual clouding of the lens often noticeable by or before 10 years of age. Since they seldom go totally blind before departing from natural causes, it usually isn't a serious problem. Surgery is an option in extreme cases but the cost is $5000 or so. Hearing loss is often sudden when dogs get into the teens and is virtually untreatable. Sometimes it's hard to differentiate from an old animal who just decides to stop paying attention.

FEEDING TABLE SCRAPS – SHOULD YOU?

I have always held the philosophy that if it's healthy for you, it's healthy for the pet. That also means that the fats, sweets, gravies and etc... that are not healthy for you are likewise not good to feed the animals. One drawback, especially in small breeds, is that they will prefer the taste of table scraps over that of dog food and turn their nose up at the latter. They're no dummies. A compromise in this case might be to mix some scraps with pet food in order to obtain a more balanced diet. Don't feed high calorie scraps to overweight animals.

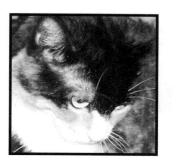

Notes

Both my dad and uncle spent their careers treating hogs and cattle and in the 40' and 50's there was a lot of physical work involved especially in regard to vaccinating hogs. They would do herds of occasionally hundreds of animals at a time and some pigs might weigh 30 or more pounds. Both men had a helper who was their constant companion and this person did most of the assisting and holding of the animals. My aunt told of one time when my uncle and helper arrived home tired and hungry. She had previously opened a can of dog food and for some reason there was a delay in feeding the animal so she put it in a bowl in the refrigerator. The hired man quickly found his way into the kitchen and made a couple of sandwiches from leftovers from the fridge. He later commented on how well he liked that new meat spread. She never had the heart to tell him what he really ate.

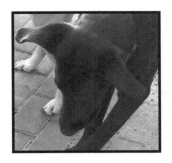 # Chapter 24

HOUSE BREAKING A DOG

Having personally house broken over a dozen dogs in my life, I can speak with a little experience. The basic principle is always the same: it has to be unpleasant for the animal if a mistake is made and rewarding when done right. My best method requires spending a few days to a week getting it used to a leash so it doesn't fight when pulled. Then when it makes a pile or puddle in the house, attach the leash, lead it to the site of the mistake, step on the leash firmly so its nose is held about four inches away and, while cleaning up, scold and shame the animal and rub some on its nose. This has worked wonderfully for me with a minimum of abuse to the animal.

Don't expect miracles too young. Some owners get the job done as early as 8 weeks of age but I have always waited until it was 12 weeks. Be reasonable in your expectations. Take it out the last thing at night, go with it and praise it when it goes outside. Get up before it does in the morning so you can also take it out in a timely fashion. Don't leave an un-housebroken pet alone in the house all day and expect it to not leave messes. This isn't realistic nor is it fair to the animal. Be persistent when you start. Some I've trained in a day and others have taken a week or more before I could trust them.

The best investment I've ever made is an all weather dog door. And living in northern Minnesota, commercial doors just didn't do a good job of holding up and keeping frigid air out. If you can find a worn fur coat at some second hand store "cheap", it will make an excellent liner. And nothing beats cow hide for the flaps. Two flaps of leather with a fur section between for insulation and fur on the sides of the frame for sealing out the cold had made an unbeatable and durable combination. I probably have the only mink lined dog door in the state. I don't tell anybody how worn and moth eaten the coat was before I cut it up.

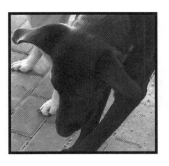

Notes

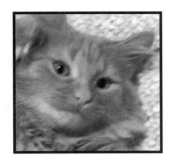

Chapter 25

CUTTING HAIR

All hair will grow back. Some people think that they shouldn't clip the hair from around some dog's eyes. Why, I do not know. The rumor that the dog will go blind is far out and unfounded. Any animal can be literally clipped down to the skin without harm and they are a lot cleaner and cooler in the summer. It will all grow back by fall. I have never known an animal to sun burn following close shearing. If you accidentally cut the skin during a clipping session, it will be categorized as minor in the realm of injuries. Small wounds will heal uneventfully in a week or so. Super glue, as strange as it may seem, will hold a flap in place to speed healing. Get the liquid—not the gel. You have to wait until any bleeding stops before applying. It is a marvelous way to stop the pain and speed healing when you have a painful crack on your finger tip or a small paper or knife cut. I keep a tube handy all the time to treat myself. If you use it to close a small flap cut on a pet, apply it to just the edges and hair. It doesn't hurt to get it on the wound itself, but try to just seal the edges together.

A client brought a Golden Retriever in one time with a fifty cent sized wound just beneath one ear. It was a fresh, clean, circular area totally devoid of skin. I asked him if he had been cutting any clumps of hair off the animal recently. He said that he had clipped some just the evening before. I told him I thought he had gotten a little too close. He didn't have any comment but a few stitches to close what was really a minor wound and he was out the door. An hour later the phone rang and it was him. He admitted he hadn't believed he could have clipped the skin without the animal showing some sign of pain so he went home and fished around in the waste basket. Sure enough there was a clump of hair with the piece of skin attached.

If you cut mats of hair on dogs and especially cats, don't pull up on the mass and try to cut under. This will nipple up the skin and you might do the same thing he did. Rather than trying to cut under mats, hold the scissors up right, gently work the pointed end under the mat and cut it into quarters or smaller pieces. Then it should comb out quite easily and not leave a bald spot. This method will work on most reasonable sized mats. The biggest ones will just have to be very carefully undermined a little bit at a time.

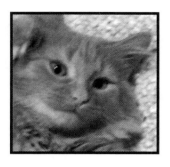

Notes

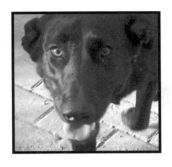

Chapter 26

CHERRY EYE

This is the term for a suddenly appearing, small, flesh colored, cherry shaped object in the inner corner of an eye. The vast majority occurs in cockers but I've seen them in many breeds. It is nothing more than a tear gland that for some reason slips out of place. They don't blind the animal but look weird. Once there, they are permanent and will darken with time. There are two ways to fix the problem.

The simple method is for a veterinarian to just clip it off and be done with it. I have probably removed at least a hundred this way without any complications of a "dry eye". Supposedly a lack of tears due to removal of the gland can result in this condition, but I have never encountered this in 40 years. This gland obviously isn't the only source of tears. The more modern and expensive way is to return it to its original location. Since I have never encountered any problem correcting with simple removal, I would be hard pressed encouraging you to spend a lot more money paying for the other method. Once removed they won't return but could show up in the other eye.

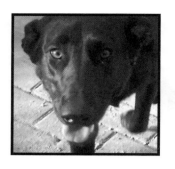

Notes

_____

_____

_____

_____

_____

_____

_____

_____

_____

_____

_____

_____

_____

_____

_____

_____

_____

_____

_____

_____

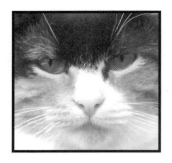 # Chapter 27

COMMENTS ON SPAYING AND NEUTERING

Spaying is an ovarian-hysterectomy (ovary/uterus removal) on a female. Neutering is removing the testicles on a male. About the only control you have over this is who does the surgery, how old the animal is when it's done and how much is spent on presurgical screening. Up to a point, the more experience the veterinarian has, the more satisfactory the outcome will probably be. This is considered a high expectation surgery meaning people assume the outcome to always be successful. No surgery is without risk.

The younger and "greener" the veterinarian, the less experience this person will have. Ask who is going to do the surgery and this person's years of experience. The newer hired, less experienced veterinarians are the ones who usually get delegated to do the "routine" surgeries.

The best time is at 4½ to 6 months of age. There is generally the least amount of complications and the animal should be up and hopping that evening. Dog neutering carries a lot more risk than spaying for several unexplainable reasons. Mature male dogs, esp. of the larger breeds, are at more risk with intravenous anesthetics when they reach or pass a year of age. Females, young dogs and other older neutered dogs don't seem to have this problem.

Atropine, if given 10 minutes before the anesthetic, has prevented this problem 100% for me so hope your veterinarian is aware of this fact. This is knowledge that comes from experience which I feel is much more important than presurgical testing. (See also chapter 11—presurgical testing)

This same group of male dogs (one year old or older) also carries a great risk of life threatening complications following the neutering. Do not ask me why but apparently a blood clot can form 48 to 60 hours following the surgery. This can happen in any male dog (never had it happen to a female) but Collies are an extreme risk. DO NOT NEUTER A COLLIE THAT IS OVER 7 OR 8 MONTHS OLD—THE RISK IS EXTREME. I have had no trouble doing it before that age.

Newfoundlands may be a similar risk. I have never seen anything written about this in the literature but trust my 40 years of experience that I know what I'm talking about. A blood thinner like aspirin plus an anti-inflammatory like prednisone seem to help prevent this from happening in any breeds except the two mentioned above. I would administer them daily for three days following the surgery. Neutering your dog young is the safest time. Cats have never been a problem at any age.

WHAT IS THE BEST REWARD

I have seen a lot of suggestions about giving your pet a small treat as a reward for doing well during a training session. I have never been a fan of this method. I spend a lot of time with my dogs and they usually accompany me whenever I'm outside. I never try particularly hard to train in any specific way but they are expected to stay within sight and come on command. The best reward, in my experience, is honest praise. Sometimes just a verbal scolding will elicit such a pained expression in their eyes that I have almost felt guilty. If you develop any kind of close relationship, they will try very hard to please and will be overjoyed just with petting and honest praise.

Many times over the years pet owners have delayed spaying a cat or dog to "allow" the animal to have a litter first. Whatever your reason, always keep this in mind: It does not make the animal more quiet and settled. There is no research to substantiate this and I have never felt anything in my forty years of owning and spaying animals gave it any credence. Unless you have a GOOD reason to bring in another litter, don't. I think I've read that some where in the neighborhood of 4 or 5 million dogs and cats are euthanized yearly in this country because no one wants them. Due to the high price of veterinary care, this number is only going to increase. Don't add to it.

One last input on spaying: Many feel it contributes to the dog taking on extra weight as a result of the surgery. I personally feel that the same dog, if it was not spayed, yet fed just as much but not allowed to get pregnant, would get just as fat. Producing and nursing puppies is the big difference in keeping its weight down. Nor do I feel it will change the dog's personality. It will be the same dog but without puppy making ability.

The advantage of neutering a dog is it will not run off chasing the fairer sex (it still might run off to do the garbage can route), it won't pee on every bush and shrub, and probably won't be quite as dominate and aggressive. Hopefully it will reduce the tendency to pick a fight and be less apt to bite both man and beast.

132

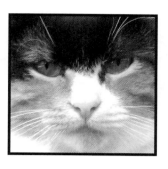

Notes

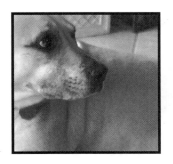

Chapter 28

WHAT ABOUT WORMING

Most veterinary establishments will require a fecal check before administering or dispensing worming medication. This is another added on fee. A negative fecal exam is NO guarantee your animal is free of parasites and shouldn't be mandatory before giving routine worming. Remember, one of the reasons veterinarians gave to justify your administering heartworm preventive year around was because it also contained pyrantel, which treated and prevented intestinal worms. In this case they wanted you to worm your animal every month without testing so they could sell more product!

You can purchase over the counter wormers if you want to routinely worm your animal. Pyrantel is probably the best one available. Large animal formulations of this wormer are available that are much more concentrated and much less expensive when worming large numbers of dogs. The higher concentration makes them much easier to give because the volume is so reduced. It's usually marked for horses and comes in a liquid (not paste) concentration of 50 mg. per ml. One ml would worm a 10 lb. animal. Worming several times a year is a good idea. The more animals you have, the more frequently you should worm. Monthly is a good idea if you raise large numbers of dogs or cats. Ivermectin is a very inexpensive wormer and the dose was previously explained in the heartworm section. It does carry a very small risk whereas I have never heard of a problem with pyrantel. Ivermectin has never been recorded to be toxic to cats, that I'm aware of, at the worming dose. 1/10th ml per 10 lbs. is the worming dose of the 1% large animal product. Don't use on collies or herding dogs with four white feet at any dose except for heartworm prevention which is 1/10th ml for 100 lbs. Any dose that strong or stronger will of course prevent heartworm infection.

You will seldom see evidence of intestinal worms but sometimes the dog or cat will throw some up or pass a few rectally as a consequence of diarrhea. THE WORM IS PASSED BECAUSE OF THE DIARRHEA AND IS NOT THE CAUSE OF IT NOR IS IT THE CAUSE OF THE VOMITING. The worm you will see would be angleworm shaped, white and the diameter of the lead in a lead pencil. This is commonly called a round worm and is treated with the above mentioned wormers. I have never known worms to cause an adult dog to act sick. I don't know how many times someone has wormed their dog because it acted off in some way.

The other worm which is commonly seen is a tape worm. Here small, white, half inch, moving segments will be noticed around the rectum or on a fresh bowel movement. These are actually not worms but tiny pieces that break off daily from the end of the tapeworm. Their sole purpose is to spread microscopic eggs around that a rodent has to inadvertently eat. The worm will then develop into the next stage in the rodent and remain there until some carnivore catches it. If the rodent is eaten by a dog or cat, the tapeworm then develops. Tapeworms can't be given from one dog or cat to another. They can only be acquired by eating an infected rodent. Only medication specific for tapeworms will rid the animal of the problem. They are not life threatening but are certainly repulsive when present. Raw rabbit is the best source for dogs. Only the cats that eat what they catch get into trouble. You will probably have to get this medication from a veterinarian and you will likely have to bring your animal in for an "exam" before being given the treatment which is just a simple pill. One type of tapeworm is spread through the ingestion of fleas, but in my northern area this is extremely rare.

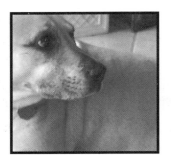

Notes

_____
_____
_____
_____
_____
_____
_____
_____
_____
_____
_____
_____
_____
_____
_____
_____
_____
_____
_____
_____
_____
_____

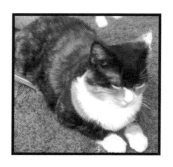

Chapter 29

VOMITING IN CATS AND DOGS

Every animal is going to throw up on occasion and it is usually nothing to worry about. Treat vomiting the same as simple diarrhea. It is often a consequence of eating too much of something upsetting to the animal. If the animal is acting really sick, a medical opinion might be warranted. If it just throws up a few times without any other noticeable symptoms, give it 24 to 36 hours as the vast majority of cases will self correct. If cats are more than three years old and long haired, throwing up RECENTLY eaten food on a regular basis is often a sign of hairballs. COUGHING IS NOT A SIGN OF HAIRBALLS. Hairball medication would be worth a try first. Vaseline is supposed to do the same thing if you can get the cat to consume about a teaspoon of it daily for several days.

Dogs will eat grass on occasion. I do not know the reason for this craving but may be they are trying to eat healthy (essential greens)! The worst that can happen as a result is throwing it up on the carpet which they seem to prefer over tile or linoleum.

COUGHING IN CATS AND DOGS

Almost all acute coughing situations are nothing more than a simple upper respiratory irritation or infection in the same realm as you would experience if you had a cold or flu. Retching up or vomiting some white phlegm is often associated with and follows the cough. If the animal is coughing severely and not eating, antibiotic is probably indicated. You can try any liquid cough medication you use on the kids but I read recently that they weren't as effective as simple sugar water. That would at least taste a lot better. Don't get into expensive testing again without just cause. Try a simple broad spectrum antibiotic like amoxicillin for a few days first. Again—save the expensive heroics for the severe unresponding cases. If it is caused by a virus, the animal will just have to wear it out like you would a cold. As long as they keep eating and drinking it isn't particularly serious. Pain medication may help.

PORCUPINE QUILLS

Do not cut the quills off. This just makes them shorter and more likely to get buried beneath the skin where they can't be reached. It DOES NOT make them pull easier! This is the epitome of old wives tales. I have probably pulled quills from a thousand dogs so I don't get too excited about seeing a few stuck in a dog's face. Removing them is simply a matter of grasping them with a pliers or forceps and pulling. Don't get paranoid about a half dozen or so because it does not constitute an after hours emergency. Having seen dozens of dogs get them repeatedly (some as often as 8 times) I don't feel too sorry for most of them. Restraint of course is the key. If you can hold the animal down and pull them yourself, you can probably save hundreds of dollars. No animal is going to die from 20 or 30 if you can't afford to pay for removal. The animal is obviously going to be regretful for a few days but it may be incentive to keep it from happening again. And don't lose any sleep over a few that might break off or be unpullable. Nature has made them pretty inert--wild animals suffer their stupidity on their own. They almost NEVER become infected. It's not unusual to see a dime sized lump develop in the lip or on the face following a quill episode but it never seems to bother the dog and eventually disappears. Don't be spooked with a little blood while pulling. It will stop uneventfully.

FOOT PAD CUTS

It is not unusual for dogs to step on something sharp, slicing a pad open and sometimes even clear off. This of course causes pain and the animal favors that particular leg. This can look bad and be painful to the dog but in the realm of injuries it is minor. It doesn't need to be stitched nor even wrapped. I don't think I have ever seen one get infected. It has an excellent chance of healing in spite of what you do so don't blow the rent money on fixing it. Within a week even the worst ones should show dramatic improvement. Sometimes, if the cut extends between the pads, a fairly large blood vessel can be severed that might require a stitch to stop persistent bleeding. A wad of cotton pressed into the area and the whole foot wrapped snugly with gauze or something similar may be adequate to stem bleeding of that nature. It would be worth a try especially if finances are short before resorting to professional help. Leave the wrap on for a day or two if possible and then just a light covering for a few days will help keep the animal from reopening the cut to cause more bleeding. A simple pad wound will NOT result in a serious bleeding problem and does not need to be wrapped. Bleeding would only be a problem if the cut extends into the hollow between the pads. This is a situation where pain medication could be a detriment. You don't want the animal walking on it or bleeding may reoccur. Soreness in this case is your ally.

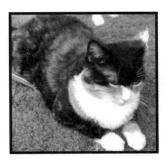

Notes

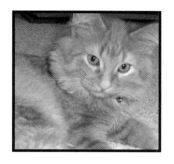

Chapter 30

HOTSPOTS AND ALLERGIES

Large dogs, especially in hot weather, will sometimes develop an acute, local, hive-like area of intense itching, where the hair will become wet and matted and sometimes even disappear. These hot spots can appear anywhere on the sides or upper body and head. They never seem to develop on the legs or underside. It just appears as a large, oozing sore. It is an allergic reaction to some unknown cause. The size can range from one inch to 4 or 5 inches across. They are usually a once in a life time occurrence. The condition responds rapidly to simple oral cortisone (prednisone) and treatment usually doesn't have to exceed a week. If the animal can lick the area, topical treatment is probably not worth while. Do NOT spend money running tests or under go allergy testing. Keeping the dog out of water for a week is important. Antibiotic is almost never indicated. If the dog simply leaves it alone, it will get better. If money is short, it will not kill the animal and will eventually be self resolving. Pain medication or antihistamines might help relieve the animal's intense itch.

Generalized allergies are common and here too the dog will start scratching on some or all areas of the body. These too are usually a warm weather occurrence and should only need a few weeks of treatment. Allergies seem to be an adult dog problem. If a puppy develops an intense itch, mange is almost always the reason. Other things can cause itch on adult dogs but, if finances are short, simply treating with the steroid prednisone for several weeks would be the place to start. If your dog's problem is a simple, seasonal allergy, this will be all that's needed. If the problem is something more complicated, the condition will persist and then decide if you can afford to spend the money to get to the bottom of it.

Again antibiotics are almost never needed. I wouldn't even consider changing diets unless you have an unusual, chronic problem. There again, most veterinarians hate to use prednisone and will give all kinds of reasons why it is not a good idea. (I've often wondered if it was too easy and successful of a treatment and it cut out the income from more involved testing and medication). Try the simple approach first and save the expensive heroics for the unresponsive cases. I've used prednisone on thousands of animals in my 40 years and I have never had a serious problem. For long term use, every other day administration is recommended, but each animal is different and it has to be used to effect. I personally know a woman client with lupus (an auto immune disease) that has been on 20 mg. of prednisone a day for 30 years so I don't consider it any more dangerous than any other human prescription drug and it probably has fewer side effects than most. A few dogs urinate more frequently when on this steroid, so morning administration in these cases will make the problem livable. If your dog can't tolerate it, then you will have to go to plan B, which will be much more expensive.

There is one type of mange (sarcoptic) that can affect adult dogs. This is something that can be difficult to diagnose. It is caused by a tiny mite that gets in the hair follicle and lives. The condition will start on the belly and legs and eventually spread

146

over the entire body. If you have two or more dogs that start itching within weeks of each other, this would be very significant because it's contagious. Allergies are not contagious. It can affect people and appear as tiny red spots on the skin. It's self curing on people and will only last a week or so. It's most common where dogs run loose, which is not the case in most communities any more. If you have a dog diagnosed with sarcoptic mange, all the dogs in the household need to be treated simultaneously plus any neighborhood dogs your pet plays with. Ivermectin at about 1 ½ times the intestinal worming dose (explained in heartworm section) given twice weekly for a month or two is effective. The animal will continue to itch for 10 days following start of treatment but should be over the symptoms by 14 days. Revolution applied on the back is also effective.

Demodectic mange, which is a problem only within a single litter of puppies, is not contagious to other dogs (or people) and is treated with ivermectin at THREE times the intestinal worming dose daily for three months. This type of mange is a puppy problem and only occurs in a litter born to a carrier mother. The other type (sarcoptic) can affect any age dog (very contagious).

Do not automatically assume an itching dog has fleas. DON'T spend money on flea products unless you actually see signs of their presence on the dog. They are pin head sized bugs, dark in color and most visible where the hair is thinnest as on the belly of the dog. Parting the hair on the lower back in front of the tail is an area they concentrate. If you see what appear to be numerous pepper flake-like specks in this area, this would be very suspicious of fleas. You use the same thing to treat for fleas as you do to prevent them. Once again, treat ALL animals in the household or you won't solve the problem. A dog with flea allergy will itch much more severely than a non allergic dog and will concentrate the biting on the flanks and back of the thighs. Getting rid of the fleas will end the allergy.

Ringworm (just for the record) is almost nonexistent in dogs (I may have seen it only on 2 or 3 litters of young puppies in 40 years), but can be a problem in cats, although it is uncommon here also. It appears as a hairless, dime or quarter sized spot that may be reddish at first but evolves into a white, crusty area. Children are ten times more apt to catch it from the animal as are adults. Systemic treatment is about the only way to go and all cats should be treated in the household. I've seen it on hundreds of 300 to 500 pound calves in NE Nebraska in the late winter/early spring when I practiced there in the 1970's. It would invariably disappear without treatment as soon as the animals got on fresh pasture. Obviously, in that case, it was related solely to nutrition. I have seen inexperienced veterinarians call Buffalo gnat bites, ringworm. Here you will see dozens of dime sized, circular, red rings with a small spot in the center, suddenly appear on dogs for just a week or so in hot weather. It seems to affect only outside dogs on the belly, where the hair is thinnest. Dogs never seem to know it's there and the bites disappear in a week whether it's treated or not. These are the same insects that will bite you under the hairline, collar or cuff that will itch for a week.

Based on the fact that I virtually never see ringworm on adult dogs and skin specialists at the University of Minnesota that I have conversed with say the same thing, if your veterinarian diagnoses it on your dog---get a second opinion from someone who's experienced.

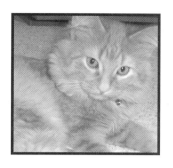

Notes

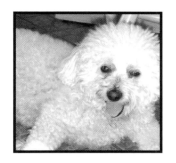

Chapter 31

BOTTOM SCOOTING

Every dog I've ever had has at one time or another scooted its rear on the carpet on an occasional basis. One used to do it at least twice a week. He preferred to perform when company was present. This would be considered a somewhat repulsive but normal behavior. If an animal suddenly makes a production out of it and does it repeatedly over a short period of time, this would indicate a minor problem. Many immediately think of worms as a cause but almost always I have found the reason to be a skin rash, irritation or local allergy in the area around the rectum. You could try any topical cortisone repeated several times a day and see if that corrected the problem before incurring an office visit. It's not serious. Just an itch to the animal and scooting is a way of scratching it. Infected anal glands hurt and the animal would not likely be rubbing its bottom on the floor. Overly full or impacted glands could possibly cause an increase in occurrence of scooting.

ANAL GLANDS

Both dogs and cats have anal glands. The two glands are located under the tail with one on each side of and level with the bottom of the rectum. They are kind of a weak cousin to a skunk's scent glands. They really serve no necessary purpose in pets and are seldom a problem. If an animal is frightened, it can squirt some of the contents out resulting in a definite "eye opening" aroma. Fortunately it washes off with soap and water and is much less challenging to remove than skunk spray. The contents of the glands are usually a thick, brown, fluid. Only on rare occasions do the glands become impacted and have to be emptied manually. This basically is no more complicated than using tips of the thumb and fore finger to gently pinch together in front of the glands (both simultaneously) and then bringing the flat part of the two fingers slowly together to force the contents out. (How hard to pinch---just hard enough to express the contents). A piece of cotton or tissue between the hand and the rectum will help catch the fluid but trust me when I say it washes off easily. A holder needs to restrain the animal just like described in nail clipping only here the animal needs to be standing and not laying.

Rarely can the glands become infected and here you will see a nasty, red swelling just below and to one side of the rectal opening. It will be very sore to the touch. It is a small abscess and will open of its own accord to let the infection drain out. It is somewhat like a bite abscess in cats. The dog will run a fever for a few days and not act up to par. When the gland breaks open, it is pretty much on the mend but antibiotics are still a good idea. If the antibiotics are given early enough, the infection shouldn't even progress to the point of breaking open. Don't let the treatment get any more involved than just a week's worth of antibiotics plus pain medication of your choice. I wouldn't recommend their removal unless you had a chronic or a reoccurring problem. Just keeping antibiotics on hand in this case and starting treating at the first sign of a problem is much simpler.

SKUNK TREATMENT: Pint of hydrogen peroxide, plus 1/4th cup baking soda and a teaspoon of liquid detergent. Massage into area for 5 minutes and rinse with water.

HERNIAS IN PUPPIES

There are two kinds of hernias that are fairly common in new born or newly acquired puppies (cats don't seem to be troubled with this as much). A hernia is either classified as an inguinal or an umbilical hernia.

INGUINAL means it is located in the rear of the crease where the hind leg joins with the belly.

UMBILICAL means where the belly button is located (umbilical cord).

Almost all are small and will NOT need to be corrected. Do not rush into surgery which is the policy of many veterinarians. The hernia, unless it's the size of a nickle on a small dog or little bigger on a larger breed will not be a health threat to the animal and even then complications would be very remote. In 40 years I have seen many hundreds and have never know one to be a problem to the animal unless it was still present as an adult and the animal went into labor. Small inguinal hernias usually are only fat and will disappear in a month or two. The tiny opening in umbilical hernias will close in similar amount of time but the bump will remain. Pinching it will result in its deflation in the young animal. When the hole closes in a month or two, it no longer will collapse when squeezed and then it's no longer considered a hernia. The bump will NOT hurt the dog but, if it's on a female, she just won't look good in a bikini.

Rushing into surgery, unless you are someone selling puppies and need correction before a sale, will usually result in spending a lot of money on something that will be self correcting if just left alone. If it never gets any bigger than a dime, forget it. With hold surgery until the animal is at least 5 months old. Then you won't get suckered into unnecessary surgery.

LICE ON PUPPIES

Very rarely I will see lice on litters or newly acquired puppies. They are usually on the back and appear as almost whitish, transparent bugs that move very slowly and are pinpoint (not pin head) sized. They are usually a consequence of the animal coming from a tough environment and are of no particular health threat. Worming the animal, good food, a bath (flea or tick is optional as they are easy to get rid of) and they seem to fade into the background. I never see them on the majority of well cared for puppies. It seems like the pup has to be in a run down condition for the mites to thrive. It's not necessary to spend a mint getting rid of them. Any flea or tick remedy seems to work. Probably just a good scrubbing or two will suffice.

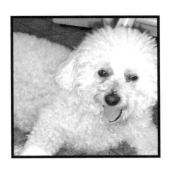

Notes

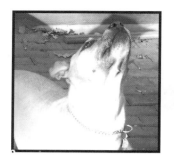

Chapter 32

DRY OR MOIST NOSE

A dog's nose can be either moist and cool or dry and warm. Both of these conditions can occur in a normal, healthy animal. Probably, if the animal was running a fever, the nose would be more likely to be dry but if the animal is acting normal, don't worry about the nose.

SEIZURES

Seizures can be quite frightening when witnessed for the first time but fortunately are almost nowhere near as serious as when they occur in people. Few dogs drive or operate heavy equipment so about the only time a seizure would be serious is when swimming. An occasional occurrence is really NOT a big deal! In dogs they can occur at any age but are basically an adult problem.

They usually appear as a staggering, progressing into where the animal falls over and stiffens out. Vomiting, urinating and defecating occur in full blown cases. If the animal is up and basically back to normal in 10 minutes, this is the normal sequence and not worth a rush to the doctor. Arriving at the clinic with a, by now, "normal animal" will only result in paying for a series of tests that will almost never detect anything. Since you can't predict when they will occur, you simply have to let a pattern get established and assume that this will be a map of the future. A seizure every month or so is probably something that isn't worth treating. When it's necessary to treat is basically a judgment call.

Generally if they happen several times a day or even weekly or last much longer than described above, I would recommend putting the animal on a preventive. The most economical preventative is phenobarbital given at an appropriate dose AM & PM. Of course, before most veterinarians will prescribe this, a thorough exam will have to be performed. Required testing will also be mandated before refilling prescriptions. There is NO legitimate reason for testing phenol levels. Apparently they figure you are not capable of recognizing if your animal experiences an occasional seizure during treatment. If a mild one does occur on rare occasion, you can increase the dosage or ignore it as not particularly detrimental to the dog, as very few will be old enough to have received their driver's license. The drug manufacturer says there is a SLIGHT chance of liver problems with chronic use. If your veterinarian states testing is necessary, ask why it is done very rarely on people. You are again at the mercy of the doctor. You will either let them run some basically unnecessary tests, or they will refuse to refill the prescription. They will readily let your animal go without medication if you won't let them get you for a fee on tests.

Animals can still have a possible seizure when on the twice a day preventative but it greatly helps lessen and prevent their occurrence. Excitement seems to trigger them so if you have a lot of company and extra noise over a weekend, giving the phenobarbital three times a day during this time might be a good idea. When people have seizures, a lot of effort and expense is spent looking for brain tumors, aneurisms, and etc. This isn't done in dogs. The cause is almost never determined in animals. Don't waste your money on expensive testing.

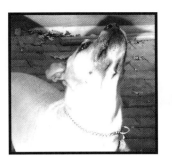

Notes

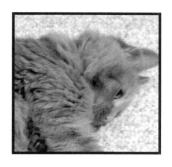

Chapter 33

DECLAWING

This can be a debated subject between lots of people but I've done thousands and consider it a worthwhile procedure. If you have a cat that scratches you or the furniture and want to keep the cat and eliminate the problem, it is the solution. It's best when done at 10 or 12 weeks of age but can be performed on any age animal. You can clip the nails with a fingernail clipper and remove the sharp points but this will not totally prevent slow destruction of furniture upholstery from a persistent animal. They may even devote more energy trying to resharpen their nails! The clipping needs to be done every several weeks. Gluing blunt balls over the animal's claws sounds more humane but most people tire of the procedure after a while. If declawing is done right, it is a pretty simple surgery. I've had cats both ways and I prefer the declawed variety by a long shot! And they can go outside and even climb a small tree. Just declaw the front feet.

Removing dewclaws and tails on puppies is BEST done when 2 to 5 days old. They can be removed at any age but, the older the animal, the more expensive and drastic the procedure will become. I would recommend removing any rear dewclaws present but all dogs have front ones and these are a normal, functioning claw. Contrary to the popular opinion of hunting dog owners, the front dewclaw doesn't get torn nearly as often as any of the other four nails do and I've seen a lot of torn nails. They seem to have a hang up on insisting the front dewclaws are removed.

PUPPIES AND TUMMY RASH

Many newly acquired 8 week old puppies have a noticeable skin condition on their tummies. It can appear as pimples, rash, tiny sores or whatever. I have seen thousands and I have never seen a condition so bad that the puppy was even aware there was a problem. It has invariably gone away without doing anything but keeping it clean and giving it adequate food and shelter. Don't waste any money on treating it UNLESS the animal acts like it's a bother.

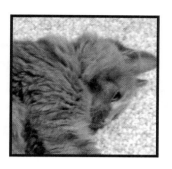

Notes

My father and uncle were large animal veterinarians and, although they both always had dogs, rarely did either one treat a dog or cat. When you consider the overwhelming deluge of veterinary care that is pushed on the animals today, it's amazing how any survived in those earlier times! Makes on wonder if all this is really necessary. Being quite young, I vaguely remember one thanksgiving when the families got together for a holiday meal. The customary turkey had come out of the oven and had been placed on the table in the kitchen to cool a little before serving. Everyone was gathered in the living room for a few minutes. My uncle had a large male Chesapeake at the time and it came trotting into the room with the whole turkey in its mouth. The turkey was retrieved, the dog caught hell and we all sat down and had our holiday meal. No one ever gave it a second thought. It always made a good story.

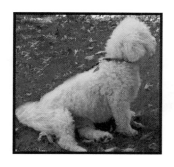

Chapter 34

MALE DOGS – PUSS FROM THE PENIS

Unneutered especially large breed male dogs can appear to drip what appears to be a greenish or yellowish puss from the end of the penis sheath. I have seen this numerous times over the years and I can't remember a dog that was ever bothered by it or affected from it. It has always been self resolving in a week or two. If it appears to be a real problem especially if the animal is irritated, have it checked out. If isn't bothering anything but yourself, give it some time and it will almost certainly disappear in a week or so.

WHEN IS AN ANIMAL RUNNING A FEVER

Many clients arrive with a pet and are sure it is running a temperature because it feels warm to the touch. Remember that dogs and cats have a normal temperature that is often several degrees warmer than humans have. A sleeping pet will awaken in the morning and have a normal temperature of 99 to 100 degrees. Average during the day is 100 to 101 degrees. Hard play on a warm day could bring it up to 103 and it would still be considered normal. In the morning 103 would be a definite fever. A thermometer inserted rectally to a depth of at least an inch and left for 60 seconds will give an accurate reading. Trying to take a pet's temperature orally is NOT a good idea! Lubricate the thermometer before inserting.

URINE LEAKING

A very low percentage of spayed dogs can sometime, later in life, develop urine leakage especially while sleeping. This is the result of a total lack of female hormone due to ovary removal. The hormone is apparently necessary for muscle control of the urethral opening. It is very easily corrected by the administration of diethyl stilbesterol at a rate of 1 mg. per 30 pounds of weight. The starting dose is once daily for four days to see if the problem is corrected and then only once weekly for maintenance. This is a far superior treatment over any of the modern replacement drugs. A veterinarian can obtain it through a compounding pharmacy. The modern way is to run the usual barrage of tests first to "determine" if that is the problem. The simpler way is to administer the drug mentioned above, see if it works, and if not, then run the more expensive tests. It is virtually 99% effective for this problem. Save the tests for the 1% that doesn't respond. A very few animals will require the weekly dose to be given oftener, like every 4 or 5 days. And, of course, before the prescription will be refilled every so many months a thorough exam will be mandatory.

The very few male dogs that have leaked urine while sleeping have had a bladder infection and responded to appropriate medication. Urine dribbling in a new puppy is usually involuntary and caused by excitement or intimidation. The animal will grow out of the problem but it may take months or longer. The dog can't help it so scolding will only make the situation worse.

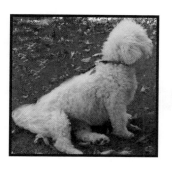

Notes

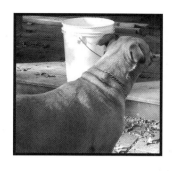

Chapter 35

TEARDROP EAR

Anatomically an ear is just a thin layer of flexible cartilage covered by two layers of skin. Sometimes, due to pinching or violent shaking, the skin can become torn away from the cartilage. This creates a potential space that the body then fills up with bloody serum. It's the same as when you pinch your skin with pliers and create a blood blister. Most occurrences are in dogs with long, hanging ears. It often starts off as a small, localized swelling that is irritating to the dog. This causes increased head shaking, spreading the swelling to eventually evolve the whole ear and thus giving the "teardrop" appearance.

There are several options:

    a. If the swelling is noticed before involving the entire ear, putting a plastic hood (explained in 37) over the dog's head to prevent shaking or a snug fitting head band with the ear over the top of the head (if the animal tolerates it) would probably prevent further progression and the small amount of fluid would reabsorb in a few weeks. You could even try taping the ear over the head. I like to administer prednisone also to minimize inflammation and help stop shaking.

    b. If the whole ear is involved, it will not kill the animal but will be a source of irritation for several weeks. It will eventually reabsorb but will take several months to completely go away and the ear will be somewhat knurled in appearance. The dog will lead a normal life but have the ear of an ex prize fighter.

c. Surgical correction involves the expense of having a dime sized hole cut in the underside skin, having the ear taped over the head for several weeks plus wearing the plastic hood (explained in 37). Some vets will even stitch it. It can be quite an involved process. If it works out, the ear should have a pretty much normal appearance. It's what you want or can afford to pay for.

Sometimes the basic cause was head shaking due to an external ear infection. This should be addressed to prevent further problems.

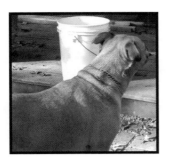

Notes

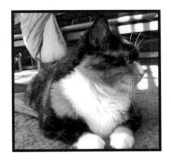

Chapter 36

PARALYSIS

Any type of paralysis is pretty much beyond the control of a veterinarian to correct. Not that a skilled orthopedic surgeon might not be able to resolve the problem in SOME cases but remember 99% of veterinarians don't have those credentials and you are talking mega bucks on a long shot. Any animal that is partially or totally paralyzed will be immediately rushed into the X-ray room and for what? You already know you have a problem and the X-ray will only show the possible source of the nerve compression at best. If the veterinarian isn't skilled enough to pursue this type of specialized surgery and if you aren't willing to spend many thousands of dollars on a long shot, DON'T start the process.

As an example: I had a client bring a Chihuahua in one time with an "almost" total posterior paralysis. He had first taken it to another, larger clinic where they had gone the route with the X-rays and tests. Spinal surgery was recommended for the estimated cost of $3000 to $4000. The client, even though he dearly loved his dog and was living on disability, was tempted to proceed. He did have the good sense to question the veterinarian's experience in this area. The doctor assured him that he was qualified. He told him he had gotten to observe that type of surgery once and could also confer with another veterinarian he knew over the phone if there were any problems. The other person had supposedly done 2 or 3 such surgeries. Wouldn't you like to be on the table with this man operating on you? The man and dog were VERY lucky. An almost total posterior paralysis slowly responded to steroids and pain medication and the dog regained total mobility. Mother Nature probably deserves the most credit.

The routine treatment is heavy doses of steroids (prednisone) and possibly pain medication for a week, plus crossing your fingers. If there is any movement at all, recovery is very possible. Basically, what you have 10 days down the road is probably what the animal will live with. Dachshunds have the greatest number of posterior paralysis problems as a result of slipped discs. An animal with a total posterior paralysis will not be able to control its urine and bowel movements and would require great sacrifice on the part of the owner in maintenance and care.

ONE MORE TIME---DON'T RUSH INTO X-RAYS. THEY ARE FINE IF YOU WANT TO PURSUE SURGERY BUT A WASTE OTHERWISE AND SURGICAL BENEFITS FOR PARALYSIS ARE VERY IFFY AT BEST.

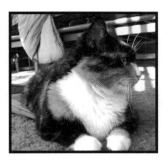

Notes

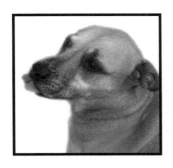 # Chapter 37

CUTS, TEARS AND BITE WOUNDS

Whether to spend money to sew up a cut or tear is often a judgment call. Almost all cuts and tears will heal with less scaring if sewn, but most small ones will heal without extra expense if just left alone. Even a 2 or 3 inch wound will probably heal uneventfully if left to nature and the dog's licking. Any wound on the front leg is a different matter. Here the animal tends to OVER lick and will keep the area from healing. Some licking is beneficial—too much is not.

In this area the restraint of a hood is necessary whether the wound is stitched or not. Wounds over joints, those with large flappy tears, and larger sized ones are better stitched. But even a 3 or 4 inch gash will potentially heal in time if money is short.

A hood (for the uninformed) is basically a large, plastic cone in the shape of a lamp shade. The small end goes around the neck and the larger end extends out past the animal's nose. It may wipe out half of the living room furniture but will keep the animal's tongue away from the area of injury.

Open cuts and gashes are not apt to get infected. Bite wounds are another matter. These animals I would highly recommend putting on a good antibiotic for 5 to 7 days.

It is common to see dime or quarter sized, raw, chapped areas on the front legs of large breed dogs. These are called lick granulomas and are the result of chronic over licking of some small sore. They don't particularly hurt anything but are unsightly. Since they are due to the habit of chronic licking, breaking the habit is the only cure. This can be a challenge. (Hoods, superglue, scolding—whatever works).

As far as self treatment of a cut or tear is concerned, anything you can do to narrow the gap will speed the body's ability to "fill in the area" so to speak. A clean, fresh wound can just be pulled together but a dirty one would best be washed. Any type of compression bandage, if the dog will allow it, will help close the area. Super glue can also be a great aid. With a large flap, just gluing the hair at the edges may cover the area and speed healing. If you can't afford to have it professionally treated, it would be the next best bet. Topical treatment with antibiotics or wound medication is usually a waste of time if the animal can lick the area. Don't make a bandage around a leg TOO tight. If you see swelling occur clear to the toes, this would be indicative of interfering with return blood flow. Just removing the bandage for a day should result in the leg returning to normal size. You would have to get it really tight for this to happen.

EYE PROBLEMS

Dogs of any age and cats (mostly adult) may suddenly develop a red and inflamed eye. With the exception of kittens, this is almost always an injury. I have never seen what I considered to be an eye infection in dogs. Kittens and very rarely more mature cats can develop an eye infection. All conditions are pretty much treated the same way. Administering an antibiotic drop or ointment several times daily for 5 to 7 days is usually all that's needed. I have always used an ointment or drop that included hydrocortisone because the benefits were much more rapid. The animal usually would be dramatically improved in 24 hours. The modern graduate will usually have this hang up about using the antibiotic including the hydrocortisone. I've used it on thousands of eyes and mine would respond much faster. I have NEVER seen a problem with the steroid. I don't know where they get those screwy ideas that cortisone is bad. I almost think they want the condition to heal slower so they can get more office visits.

If the eye is back to normal in a few days to a week, there is NO reason to pay for a follow up exam. Kittens can get either a bacterial or viral eye infection or an injury. Bacterial cases will respond rapidly to antibiotic application whereas viral will not. I ran into some cases of Herpes pinkeye lately from a humane society that were virtually untreatable. Fortunately this is rare and I hope I never see any more cases like that. Herpes is a type of virus – bad news in those cats.

The worst case scenario in an eye injury is where the cornea (the clear, front surface of eye) is gouged so deeply that the fluid behind it will start to rupture out. If a small pimple or any type of protrusion is seen on the surface of the cornea, then sewing the eyelids shut for 2 weeks has saved every eye I have ever tried it on. It's a simple procedure and has literally worked miracles in treating eyes that seemed too advanced in rupturing to even have a chance of recovery.

Short nosed, bug eyed dogs (Peks, Bostons, Pugs, etc) are most susceptible to eye injuries for obvious reasons. If one is injured so severely that the eye is sticking way out of the socket, this will almost always require complete removal. It looks absolutely terrible but does NOT constitute an after hours emergency. You will probably be a lot more distressed over it than the animal will be. If you rush it in after hours, it will be put in a cage and attended to the following day—not that night. The time frame for pushing it back into the socket seems to be very short. If the eye has been out for an hour or more, I have never been successful in returning it to its normal position and the one time I did manage to put it back, the eye was blind.

Some dogs, especially larger breeds, can develop a persistently draining eye because the edge of the lower eyelid will roll inward allowing the hair on the outside to touch the eyeball. This can occur at any age and be slight or extreme. It won't kill the animal but, once it develops, is usually permanent until corrected. Surgery to pull the lid back straight is the only solution.

*One final story that epitomizes my feeling of what the profession has become: My wife and I were relaxing at a pub one time, when another veterinarian, that I'd met once, happened by and sat down at our table for a quick chat. He was accompanied by his better half. Quite soon he offered up the information that he had recently performed spinal surgery on a client's dog. I think he was bragging because this is not a common operation. As the story unfolded, the animal had been at his hospital for several days before the client gave him the go ahead to proceed. I assume the delay was due to accumulating the necessary finances. The timing was such that the surgery was performed on a Sunday. Being willing to sacrifice his day off and operate on a Sunday impressed and gratified the pet's owner, this good doctor related. Then with his next breath he smiled and said it also enabled him to charge

more. As an after thought, he also mentioned that the owner
had waited way too long. It is my understanding that posterior
paralysis from a slipped disc needs to be corrected within 24 hours
to have much chance of success. In other words, the veterinarian
was bragging about performing spinal surgery that probably had no
benefit to the animal. The wife ended the story by remarking that
it was an easy $2500. I get angry every time I recall this incident.

It is wonderful that modern medicine enables surgical
procedures to be performed on animals that rival those done on
people. Nothing is impossible. Even transplants are performed.
This is great if you both want and can afford it. What I've
compiled in this book are my recommendations for economizing
your pet's health care. It is basically a second opinion that gives
you an informed choice between choosing the modern expensive
way, or the common sense method of doing no more than what
experience dictates is usually necessary. It comes from an old
veterinarian who has spent four decades in continuous practice
and quite a successful one at that. This information is mainly
for those who are living with restricted budgets, which seem to
be getting squeezed more with each passing year, and those who
simply don't like to waste money. A pet owner who possesses
the right information will be in a much better position to decide
intelligently. Choosing what to do based solely on emotion is very
costly in this day and age. I hope what I have written serves you
well.

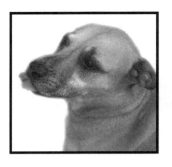

Notes

_____
_____
_____
_____
_____
_____
_____
_____
_____
_____
_____
_____
_____
_____
_____
_____
_____
_____
_____
_____
_____
_____
_____
_____
_____
_____

The Author

Dr. Busby was born on April 20, 1940 in Wayne, Nebraska. He grew up and spent his pre-college years in Wakefield, Nebraska; a small farming community in the northeast corner of the state. The first four years of higher education were at Wayne State Teacher's College. He then went four more years and received his DVM degree from Kansas State University which was where both his father and uncle also received their degrees.

After graduating in 1966, he took over his father's large animal practice in his home town and remained there until moving to Bemidji, Minnesota in 1979. There his focus turned completely to small animals (dogs and cats) and this has occupied his time for the past 26 years. He has always worked alone and has perfected his art as an outpatient practitioner.

He always gives his clients options and never hesitates to refer a patient to the university or a fully equipped veterinary hospital when necessary. He is finding that his type of services seem to be in ever growing demand in this day and age of skyrocketing animal health costs. This book is full of his experienced and common sense knowledge and will enable you to decide the type and depth of care your animal needs. I think you will find it a very valuable asset.

Purchasing Information

To order additional copies:

Send $19.95 plus $3.50 for shipping and handling. (Mail orders send check, money order or credit card information and be sure to include readable address and phone number).

Send to: Dr. Jim Busby
          Old Country Vet
          1726 Jefferson Ave SW
          Bemidji, MN 56610

Substantial volume discounts are available for purchasing the book for fund raising purposes.

Contact us for detailed information.
          www.oldcountryvet.com`

If I come across any new information that would benefit pet owners, I will list it in the "News and Updates" section of my web page. Check it occasionally.

                                        Dr. Busby